Chronic Illness and Eating Disorders

Chronic Illness and Eating Disorders addresses the intersection of eating disorders and the importance of treatment of clients with eating disorders and chronic illness, specific interventions, and resilience in a body that continues to change.

This book explores the intricacies of those with chronic illness, and how it can lead to disordered eating. Chapters cover lifelong and acquired illnesses and conditions, visible and invisible disabilities, sports injuries, chronic pain, grief, and more. The author examines how each of these conditions can affect appetite, body image, and overall perception of food and health. Treatments such as EMDR and CBT are discussed alongside mindful approaches such as body neutrality.

Therapists, dietitians, and other medical professionals will gain a deep understanding of body image disturbance and how that is different from body image distortion.

Tamie Gangloff, MA, MFT, holds a master's in clinical psychology from Antioch University in Santa Barbara. She works for a treatment center and is an adjunct professor.

"Finally, those with concurrent chronic illnesses and eating disorders have a validating piece of representation that thoughtfully, authentically, and compassionately evaluates all aspects of this complex relationship. Tamie shares her own beautiful, challenging, real story throughout, as well as others', while interpreting it through the lens of her extensive clinical experience. The result is a resource that will improve individuals', loved ones', and clinicians' understanding about how best to show up for those who have been mostly invisible to eating disorder and health care systems."

Jennifer L. Gaudiani, *MD, CEDS-C, FAED,*
is the founder and medical director of the Gaudiani Clinic and
author of Sick Enough: A Guide to the
Medical Complications of Eating Disorders

"Tamie has written a powerful resource for clinicians who work in the field of eating disorders and for anyone who lives with or knows someone who lives with a chronic disability. She gently opens the door for us to discover misperceptions we hold about living with a chronic illness to change how we interact and communicate within personal and professional settings. The reader is invited to explore the impact a chronic disability has on mental health, body image, personal relationships, professional interactions, and co-occurring conditions. Practical guidelines based on evidence-based research and lived experience are abundantly offered."

Tammy Beasley *MS RD CEDS-C,*
National Director of Nutrition Programming,
Odyssey Eating Disorder Network

"Tamie delivers an important piece of work for clinicians and clients, offering information and tips for navigating the recovery journey. Tamie covers a wide range of topics, such as weight stigma and how this can impact body image, increasing the risk of developing or perpetuating an eating disorder. Well-researched and informed suggestions are given to clinicians and clients to navigate eating and body image issues as well as several other critical areas such as embodiment, grief, resilience, medical trauma, exercise, and advocacy."

Carolyn Costin, *MA, MEd, MFT, FAED, CEDS,*
The Carolyn Costin Institute, and author of
8 Keys to Recovery from an Eating Disorder

Chronic Illness and Eating Disorders

Assessment, Clinical Skills, and Lived Experiences

Tamie Gangloff

Routledge
Taylor & Francis Group

NEW YORK AND LONDON

Designed cover image: ©Getty Images

First published 2026
by Routledge
605 Third Avenue, New York, NY 10158

and by Routledge
4 Park Square, Milton Park, Abingdon, Oxon, OX14 4RN

Routledge is an imprint of the Taylor & Francis Group, an informa
business

ISBN: 978-1-032-81530-5 (hbk)
ISBN: 978-1-032-81226-7 (pbk)
ISBN: 978-1-003-50025-4 (ebk)

DOI: 10.4324/9781003500254

Typeset in Optima
by KnowledgeWorks Global Ltd.

Contents

Acknowledgments

I am fortunate to have found medical providers who have made my world a better place. Kindness, in the midst of struggle, is what we need most. For chronic patients, like me, you need to develop long-term trusting relationships.

Dr. Mark Tantorski—you changed my life and gave me my life back. You taught me what it truly means to have a therapeutic alliance. Your kindness, compassion, expertise, and empathy have changed me, and I will forever be grateful to you. Your humaneness, understanding, and hugs are just as important as your skill as a doctor. It is because of you that I am now able to help so many others. Thank you for being a part of my E True Hollywood Story … You also still owe me a swim, even if it is in a pool with a snorkel!

Megan Cullen—your sense of humor, big smile, and hugs are just as healing as the PT. I am not the average patient, and you are not the average DPT—you are an amazing physical therapist and friend. You literally taught me how to walk again. We talked about it all—from dating to body image and everything in between. I will always remember the Turkey Trot 2019 with you! We have developed a relationship that has spanned many years. I am so blessed to have you in my life.

Dr. Jennifer Payne—you are just the best! I met you at a low point in my life, after I was injured by a medical provider. You made it easy to trust you. I feel seen and heard; I never feel dismissed or misled. I think I see you more than most of my friends! I am so thankful to have you in my corner and I love that we can have nerdy conversations about spine conferences while we address my many aches and pains. Thank you for being you (and for the mini pies!).

My twisted sister, my little big sister, Tara—you inspire me every day. You are the reason I started running and competing in triathlons, and I have so many great memories with you. I remember your support through some of the hardest times in my life, including my big surgery (and the other ones, too). During our hardest times, I couldn't imagine that we would have the friendship that we have today, and I'm so grateful and thankful for you.

Mom—thank you for always believing in me. My road has not been an easy one, and whether it was from near or far, I know that you are here for me and proud of me. You showed me what it meant to be resilient long before I understood what it meant. The time we share is the most precious gift. Love you.

The amazing humans who entrusted me with your stories—I am blessed and grateful for you! Thank you for your vulnerability and bravery, and for sharing your story so it can help others. You inspire me, and I am grateful beyond words.

My fellow warriors, mentors, and friends—this list is endless. I am beyond blessed to be on this journey with you.

My fur babies—if anyone knows me, you know that they are my heart. They have helped me through injury, surgery, and writing this book! Their love is unconditional. Rocky, Mila, Lynda Carter, Leela, and Fiona Gallagher! I lost my Rocky, my old man, recently, but don't worry … he makes a couple of appearances in this book!

My wonderful editor, Natalie Silver. You took my words and helped me create something beautiful. You talked me through my meltdowns and reminded me that I have something important to say. Your direction, support, and kindness have been invaluable to me.

Why I Wrote This Book

As an athlete with a disability, my journey through spine surgeries and the lengthy recovery process has equipped me with the tools to overcome injuries and surgeries and to navigate life in this body. While it can be unpredictable and frustrating at times, I know that I can always recover. One source of inspiration for me has been reading books by athletes who have triumphed over incredible odds after life-threatening injuries. Their stories have given me hope that I, too, can recover stronger than ever. I hope that sharing my story will inspire you with that same hope.

Throughout this book, I will share my personal experiences and some of my relevant social media posts. I have documented my journey online for several years, and I hope that this content will resonate with you.

In my research, I discovered only one study that addressed the relationship between spine surgery and mental health, which indicated that about one in five spine fusion patients experience PTSD. This finding is significant. When I face something major, I find it helpful to take action, so I created a ten-question web survey and posted it on social media. I initially expected to receive maybe 20 or 30 responses, but I was astonished to gather 185 responses. It became clear that there were voices that needed to be heard, and I felt compelled to do something with this information.

I acknowledge my privilege: I have thin privilege. I have white privilege. I am cisgender. I am heterosexual. I have health insurance. I have access to quality healthcare.

Part 1

My Story with Chronic Illness, an Eating Disorder, Substance Abuse, and Trauma

Part 1 contains my story about chronic illness and how it contributed to my eating disorder as well as years of physical and mental setbacks. My lived experience inspired me not only to write this book but to speak up on behalf of those encountering the same or similar issues as me.

Living with scoliosis has been a long, winding journey and led not only to an eating disorder in my teens and twenties but also to body image issues as a teenager, alcoholism, posttraumatic stress disorder, medical trauma, and other strains on my mental health. I want to share my story before I get into the clinical aspects of treating someone with an eating disorder who also has a chronic illness in the hope that it offers perspective on how complicated it is to live with a chronic condition and the many obstacles an individual with one (or more) encounters throughout their life. I hope you find my story resonant and that it can help you bring more understanding and compassion to your practice.

Please note, my story does describe a lot of situations that may be triggering, so please keep in mind that it includes descriptions of eating disorders, substance abuse, and suicidal behavior.

- Chapter 1: My Backstory: Scoliosis, an Eating Disorder, Alcoholism, PTSD, and Spine Fusion Surgery

DOI: 10.4324/9781003500254-1

Chapter 1

My Backstory: Scoliosis, an Eating Disorder, Alcoholism, PTSD, and Spine Fusion Surgery

Facing a Scoliosis Diagnosis at 13

I cried in the fitting room; this was the first of countless times. This was not my body in the mirror—I was in shock. This time, it was because I was sporting a new part of me, a hard plastic shell. I felt like I couldn't breathe. The brace started below my armpits, pressed into my skin, and felt intolerable. My mom and I tried to find clothes to hide my new accessory, but despite our attempts, this was just not possible. I could not take it. I would rather die than wear this anywhere, let alone in public or at school. This was my first experience in public grappling with the treatment required for my scoliosis.

Up until this moment, I had become familiar with visiting DuPont Hospital in Delaware (which is today called Nemours Children's Hospital), and it was always a positive experience. I liked the staff, the giant stuffed animals in the lobby, and the nice doctors, and I was always excited to learn which color module we would be going to do that day. I would get an x-ray of my spine, which always showed a slight curve, and then I was cleared to return in six more months.

Even at 13, I knew the horrors of scoliosis, as I had been a firsthand witness to my sister's experience with her severe curve. She was braced at a young age and needed a spine fusion as a kid. I remember having ice cream sundaes in the hospital the night before her surgery, and I also remember that it was scary for my parents and incredibly painful for my sister. I had no concept that it was possible that I would experience the same thing. I assumed that everyone else also had a slight curve in their spine, that it was normal, and that I was immune to what my sister had endured.

When doctors told me that my curve had increased to about 30 degrees and that I would need a brace, I was in shock and disbelief. My world stopped and everything went dark. This couldn't be happening to me. Being fitted for the brace was demoralizing. I was an adolescent girl wearing a cotton stockinette and getting slathered with plaster.

DOI: 10.4324/9781003500254-2

I dissociated to distract myself during this process. Dissociation was my first coping skill, and it protected me for many years. While the plaster was hardening, the technicians had to shape it, indent it, and use their fists to mold it so it would inhibit curve progression. This was then molded into my new shell and was trimmed and fitted with moleskin to prevent chafing. Watching this happen in front of my eyes felt unreal.

So that day in the dressing room, I was facing the unthinkable. I had been told that I had a deformity. *Deformity? You mean ugly, gross, and disgusting?* That's what that word meant. It's how I felt, and I always carried that word with me. I stared into the mirror, feeling grotesque in a torture device.

I couldn't fathom having to live my life in this brace. I attempted to wear it to school, and I hated how I looked and how my body felt. I couldn't sit comfortably in a chair. I was already picked on for being skinny and smart, and now I had this too! I began to refuse to wear it to school, which, of course, did not make my parents happy or treat the curvature of my spine.

My father reached out to my doctor and was told that they would cast me if I did not start to comply by wearing my brace 16 hours per day. I understood the seriousness of this, so I decided to forego it at school and put it on at home to meet the doctor's requirements. I remained devastated by having to wear this brace. This started a pattern of isolation and depression that continued for years. I did not want to go out into the world while wearing the brace, and I was very unhappy with my body because I needed to wear it. As my hatred for my body grew, so did my instinct to shrink. I wanted my body to be smaller so that nobody would notice me. I didn't want anyone to see me and how gross I was. What I knew for sure is that if they saw what I saw, they would know that I was gross and unlovable. From my adolescent perspective, no one could love a monster, and this brace made me one.

Having to wear a brace as a young teenager spiraled into so much more. I was dealing with a physical disability while also negotiating the emotional complexities of being 13 and 14. The self-consciousness started with a brace, but it evolved into issues with eating and body image, dealing with sexual trauma, and experiencing social isolation. I began to deprive myself of food during this time, and at just 14 years old, I was sexually assaulted. I was disgusted by my mushy stomach as I had lost muscle tone because the brace took away my need for core strength—it was acting as my core strength. I was at war with my body: I was shrinking it, getting weaker, and trying to be so small that I would be undetected by others. These things, combined with a family and societal culture for thinness became the perfect storm that led to my eating disorder.

My life then became a blur, and I spent these brace-wearing years in a haze. I know I missed out on a lot of time with friends. They were angry with me for not spending time with them. How could they not understand that I was sentenced to this brace, and I had no way out? I was convinced that they would not love me, my weak body, and my eroded self-esteem. I couldn't hang out, eat, or swim in their pools. I wore a long-sleeved shirt and pants to a friend's pool party because I didn't want anyone to see my uneven hips and waist as well as my withering body.

At this time, I had no tools to deal with my emotions. I felt like I couldn't breathe. My chest was tight, and I couldn't think clearly. I was one of the smart kids, yet I was not doing well in school. I was lost and didn't see a way out. I didn't want this life, but I didn't know how to say that. I had no words for my anguish. I just knew that I could not stand to be in my skin, in that body, and in this world.

Free of the Brace but Not the Baggage

After two years, I had grown enough to be discharged from wearing my brace, but my self-perception did not improve. Although I was no longer wearing the brace, I was still left with a distorted, deformed, and twisted body and did not know how to handle the emotional turmoil. I continued to sink deeper into self-loathing and did what I needed to do to avoid that pain.

When a person has scoliosis, their spine is curved from side to side and they also have a rotation in their spine called a *thoracic kyphosis*, better known as a rib hump. So, when someone with an unfused spine bends forward, you can see a hump on their back. As a teenager, I was highly conscious of my rib hump. I could feel it when I sat in a chair—only one side of my back would touch the seat. This never left my mind.

Unfortunately, my coping strategies to deal with the challenges of scoliosis did not end when doctors relieved me of my brace. I continued to rely on my new friend, one that I created during my time of seclusion from the outside world. My friend kept me thin and wanted me to stay small. My friend told me to feverishly weigh myself, check my body in the mirror regularly, and measure my waist. My real-life friends were fearful because I was so small, but I did not see that—I saw fat. A friend confronted me about my body, and I responded with a scathing reply that she was just jealous of me. This response wasn't me being a mean girl; I just did not see what she saw. I thought she was lying to me or exaggerating. I told myself there was nothing to worry about!

At the time of my adolescence, there were no words for what was happening to me, and there was no internet, so I could not dig deeper about my issues. No one spoke of eating disorders, and I certainly had no idea that I had one. There weren't easy outlets for therapy or counseling about chronic medical conditions, sexual trauma, or even just growing up. I didn't understand what was happening to me until years later.

Around the time my friend confronted me about my body size, I took my first sips of alcohol, which would be the "solution" to my low self-esteem for many years. I was at a friend's house—his dad was having a party—and we were sneaking beer upstairs. I was nervous and intrigued as I put my lips to the bottle, tipped it up, and swallowed the drink. I began to feel tipsy. This was the first time I felt the freedom that alcohol could bring. My brain indicated to me that I had found the solution to my mental struggles.

When I was drunk, I didn't feel ugly, I wasn't a nerd, I wasn't skinny, I wasn't being made fun of, I wasn't too shy to dance. When I was drunk, I could be me—I felt the most *me* I had ever felt. What I didn't realize is that I was dependent on these new friends—my eating disorder and alcohol—to continue to cope with this self-hate shadow that followed me everywhere. I could not escape it. I could only hope to hide from it by not eating and drinking.

As my life moved along into young adulthood, the medical monitoring for my scoliosis faded away. When I graduated from high school, I also felt I had graduated from scoliosis. At that time, no one told me that I needed to continue to follow up with a spine doctor. This false assumption and unconscious medical neglect would haunt me later.

I did not leave my coping mechanisms behind when I entered college (like I thought I was leaving my scoliosis), and they only magnified over time. I went to a college close enough to home but just far enough away that I felt I could be independent. Despite my initial hopes that I could reinvent myself in college, I was still so painfully shy and uncomfortable in my own skin, and I didn't like who I was. I was ashamed of my body, where I came from, and the life that I led. I didn't want anyone to know who I was.

Despite my insecurities, I began my college experience like most kids. I started to go to parties with friends and even joined a co-ed national honor fraternity, where I met lifelong friends. I also learned how to drink like a college kid—at least that's how I thought college kids drank. However, I continued to hide my eating disorder and cope by abusing alcohol. I started binging and abusing laxatives, coupled with periods of restricting food and heavy drinking.

As time marched forward, college became a blur of parties, blackouts, and lost friendships. My behavior and mental well-being were unsustainable. I had to take time off school to get help. Although I was unwilling to admit I had a problem with alcohol, I knew that I had a problem with eating and depression. No one talked about eating disorders back then, so it took some time before I knew what was wrong with me. I went to a treatment center for my eating disorder, but due to insurance, I was only able to stay for a short stint, so it was not nearly enough time to regulate my eating, emotions, and medication. The center sent me to my first 12-step meeting, and I only agreed to go because it meant I could get out of the facility for a bit. I denied that I was an alcoholic—I thought it was a big cult. Following my time in the treatment center, I did attempt to stay away from alcohol for a short period of time, but I gave up when friends brought out shots. I figured that I could partake in the fun because I didn't have a problem.

In spite of this break from school and initial treatment, my depression worsened. I remember my mom reminding me that alcohol was a depressant, and I said, "Well, I feel better when I'm drinking." I was not only in denial, but I was working so hard to avoid feeling my emotions that I could not possibly stop. My eating disorder reached new heights, leading me to the emergency room many times because my body couldn't sustain what I was doing to it. My drinking increased, and my depression went from suicidal thinking to being actively suicidal. However, I had very few resources to untangle my many issues. I knew that I did not want to live this way anymore, but all I could do was wish I could keep my eyes closed.

My life snowballed, and I no longer had any control of it. I attempted suicide. Afterward, I went back to the same treatment center. This time, I was much more beat up and much more willing to get help. When I left after a short period of time, I thought I was on the right track, finally.

Reaching Bottom and Facing New Realities

Despite the efforts to get better in college, I continued to ride the roller coaster of my eating disorder and substance abuse after graduation. I hit bottom again at 22 after a professional speaking engagement at a school where I was visibly intoxicated. I was working for a rape crisis center, which was not a great choice considering my own ignored sexual trauma that I experienced as a young teenager. I was set to talk to young kids about prevention, and there were parents there. As much as I thought I was good at hiding my substance use, I was not fooling anyone, and I got some pretty awful looks from parents during my presentation. They knew I was under the influence. I will never forget how I felt that day: out of control, unprofessional, and demoralized. It still makes me sick to think about it. Rather than returning to work following the event, I went home and started to make phone calls to get help.

I contacted seven rehab centers to get help that day. The admissions staff repeatedly said that they could not help me because I also had an eating disorder. When I talked to the last place, I told them that I knew I was not going to make it, that I was going to die if I didn't get help soon. They said that they had a counselor who knew about eating disorders, and they agreed to take me in. I went through their doors despite insurance barely covering detox. The county paid for my short stay in rehab because I could not get assistance from insurance because of my previous stint in a treatment center for an eating disorder.

Unfortunately, I still struggled with sobriety even after this moment. I did one of the things the rehab staff told me not to do. I got a rehab boyfriend, and we drank together even after getting help. Yet again, I ignored all of the signs to stop drinking until one day—May 5, 1997—the physical pain from drinking became too much. I was drinking and needed to say no to the next shot and get to the emergency room. I am grateful that I had so much physical pain from drinking that I could not continue and did go seek medical help; it truly saved my life. I have been sober ever since.

My sobriety freed me from the shackles of substance abuse, but I still struggled with restricting my food. I was able to stop using laxatives, self-harm, and some other behaviors by putting them in the same category as alcohol, but I could not overcome all of my coping mechanisms at that time.

While I continued my sobriety journey and tried to get a handle on my eating disorder, I began to experience physical pain from scoliosis at 25. At that time, my back started to hurt significantly from a short stint working in information technology where I had to lift heavy objects—computer monitors were monstrous back then! I went to the doctor, who sent me for a scoliosis study and an MRI. A scoliosis study provides a view of the whole spine in one film. It revealed a curve progression into the 40s as well as herniated discs. I felt like I had whiplash. Remember, I thought I had graduated from scoliosis when I graduated from high school. I had no idea that my scoliosis could progress in adulthood. My head spun: I wore the brace as a teenager, I stopped growing, and I was cured! This was not supposed to happen. My heart raced; I felt so afraid and alone.

Not long after this news, I stepped into the shower one day and my right leg gave out. I had awful pain down my leg, and it was numb. When I screamed, my roommate came downstairs to find me and helped me get dressed and call my dad. He had to carry me to the car, and I went to the hospital. I could not stand or walk. I had never experienced pain like this before. Following this incident, I went on disability from work and started spine injections, which had no effect. I traveled to Philadelphia to see a spine specialist, Dr. Rushton, who determined that I needed a microdiscectomy at L3/4 to manage my pain and loss of function. Following the surgery, I woke up and did not have pain down my leg. It was miraculous. I went to physical therapy and was able to go back to work but in a job that did not require heavy lifting. I needed to switch jobs to avoid straining my back again.

While I was feeling physically better from the microdiscectomy, my eating disorder was still present and getting worse, to the point that Dr. Rushton asked me about it at my follow-up appointment, where I held a Wawa coffee and had a pack of cigarettes hanging out of my purse. He point-blank asked me how much weight I had lost since the procedure.

When I tried to say that I hadn't lost any weight, he said that he could see that I had and proceeded to draw a diagram of how bones receive calcium; since I was not eating enough, he was concerned that I had osteoporosis. Dr. Rushton ordered a DEXA scan for me, which is done to check bone density. My results showed osteopenia, which meant that I had bone loss but not to the severity of osteoporosis. Furious at myself and the diagnosis, I went on a hunger strike, but not for long.

Finally Recovering from My Eating Disorder

A few weeks after this confrontation from Dr. Rushton, I reached out to an eating disorder treatment program and entered into intensive outpatient treatment. It didn't take long for the program to realize that I needed more, and I started day treatment. As I nourished myself, the feelings I had suppressed for years started to surface. My therapist, Tasha, who stayed in my life for many years, took out the DSM and reviewed the diagnostic criteria for posttraumatic stress disorder (PTSD) with me. With this diagnosis, it was like someone turned on the lights for the first time. This was it—this was me, this is what was driving that dark shadow of self-hate that followed me everywhere. Understanding the diagnosis helped me move forward and also not feel like I was crazy. For the next six months, I stayed out of work, completed day treatment, resumed intensive outpatient treatment, and continued my outpatient work.

I had never met anyone who recovered from an eating disorder— "recovered" was not in my vocabulary. One day, while I was in treatment, a woman came in to tell her story. She looked beautiful, healthy, strong, and confident as if she had a great life. When I heard her share her story, she had been just as sick as I had been with medical complications (which are not necessary to seek help), and she also struggled with feeling suicidal. If she could get better, truly better, not just white-knuckling it for a few years in between treatment stays, then maybe I could too. Upon hearing her story, I went after recovery like I never had before.

I stuck with it this time. I never looked back. I took what I learned in early recovery toward the rest of the challenges in my life. Sobriety and eating disorder recovery were not easy, but I learned how to overcome these challenges with a lot of support from others. To this day, I feel incredibly blessed and grateful for this turning point.

Scoliosis Strikes Again

When I was 29 years old, I was sober, recovered from an eating disorder, married, and living in Arizona. I was strong in my life and in my recovery. My spine, however, was not. I started to have more pain again, and it was interfering with my life. It hurt to sit for long periods of time, stand, or do most things. I realized that I needed more medical help.

I had to find a new spine doctor on the other side of the country, and I was lucky to find Dr. William Stevens. Much like my scoliosis study and MRI from several years prior, he discovered that my curve had progressed again. I was diagnosed with degenerative disc disease. My L5/S1 was severely herniated, causing pain in my back and down my legs. I knew what was next: another surgery. I was defeated and fearful; I did not want to do this again.

My second microdiscectomy was a success, and my pain improved. I also successfully recovered without retriggering my eating disorder. I was healthy and strong and pushed myself hard in physical therapy. I wanted to get strong, so I would never need surgery again. However, my resolution did not match the advice of my doctor. At that time, Dr. Stevens recommended curve correction surgery, but I said, no way—I was supposed to never need to have that surgery! I gathered my medical records from childhood and got a second opinion. The second doctor did not agree that I needed to have that surgery because the rest of my spine was stable.

For the next several years, I lived my life with varying degrees of pain and limitations. I was not an athlete back then, but I tried to exercise and walk often and stay strong. I accepted that I would always have pain in my life.

Training to Help Others with Eating Disorders

After recovering from back surgery and spending some years in Arizona, my husband and I moved to California, and not long after, I decided to go back to school. I had always wanted to help others; however, I was not equipped to do that before. Now that I had been sober for many years and recovered from my eating disorder, I knew that it was time to explore new professional opportunities. I threw myself into several opportunities. Carolyn Costin, a leader in the eating disorder recovery field and founder of the treatment center Monte Nido, held study groups at her treatment program back then. Anyone could attend, so I showed up because I wanted to learn from her. I served as a student volunteer at the National Eating Disorders Association conference that year. It was overwhelming since I was brand new to the field, but I felt a strong sense of purpose about helping others with a condition I had lived with for so many years and finally recovered from. Afterward, I enrolled at Antioch University Santa Barbara, where I had a wonderful cohort and met amazing people. I was in the right place to learn and grow.

I was able to start working for Monte Nido, and I always say that I was one of the lucky ones. I got to work for Monte Nido when Carolyn was in the program regularly. To this day, I tell everyone about my first official day of work when Carolyn asked if I wanted to sit in on her primary group. I learned from the best pioneers in the eating disorder field. Many of those people are still friends and mentors to this day.

Working in a treatment center challenged me in ways that I hadn't anticipated; it was physically demanding with long hours of sitting, standing, and helping in the kitchen. My back pain was always there, and it was a struggle. I did not have a physical therapist. I tried to take walks to get stronger, but it was hard to find the time while working and going to school. Pain was a part of me.

In addition to the challenges of work and physical pain, my marriage ended not long after graduating with my master's degree. I moved back to the East Coast, and it was time to start over. I had a rough landing back in New Jersey, but with the support of friends and family, I was able to land on my feet. Because of prior experiences, I knew I needed to get help for my depression and PTSD to deal with the changes in my life, and I did enter an inpatient unit for a few weeks.

Reinvention and Setbacks

The pain and limitations from scoliosis significantly contributed to my self-esteem as a now-single woman in midlife. I was fulfilled in my career, but I wanted more from life. I was in great shape and focused on fitness to stay strong as well as to socialize with others, but I struggled with how I looked because of the scoliosis, and I was very hesitant when it came to dating and relationships. Even though I was years recovered from an eating disorder, I still was not okay with my uneven waist and hips. I was self-conscious and ended up in relationships that were not good for me. I still felt like I was defective, just as I had at 13. This low self-esteem contributed to me being in an abusive relationship for many years.

Despite the problems in my romantic relationships, I continued to develop resilience in other ways. My sister was running and doing triathlons at this time. When we were kids, they discouraged exercise for kids with scoliosis, but they now encourage it. I wanted to try what my sister was doing, and I signed up for my first 5K. I then joined her triathlon club, bought a bike, and learned how to swim breaststroke by watching YouTube videos. Diving into the world of triathlon was truly transformational. I found a new tribe of women and found them to be hugely supportive.

My career was on the right track. Years after my move back to the East Coast, I returned to my first treatment program, with a new location in Pennsylvania, to work in outreach. I felt a huge sense of satisfaction seeing clients, connecting with other professionals, and creating eating disorder awareness events. However, during this time, my back pain was also worsening again. I returned to Dr. Rushton in Philadelphia, and he said that I looked stable and that I could continue my activity but not run long distances. I needed to focus on staying strong, which would help my bones and my overall health.

Despite this change of approach to my health and fitness, I had increasing difficulty sitting in the car for hours, which was a requirement for my job. The pain diminished my quality of life. I could not run or ride my bike, but I continued to swim. Open-water swimming was my salvation from pain and from life. I loved it, with my longest swim being a 10K in the Hudson River. I felt at peace in the water despite the physical limitations and pain I was experiencing.

Getting a Definitive Surgery

I was not free of pain in my back despite my fitness level and making accommodations in my professional life. I found a new surgeon, Dr. Mark Tantorski, to discuss treatment options. At 43 years old, my lumbar spine had no cushion left. Dr. Tantorski recommended injections for pain, which I tried for several years, and we did not discuss surgery until it became necessary. At that point, my pain was unbearable, and I lost feeling in my left foot and started to trip when I walked.

When we started to discuss surgical options, I asked if we could correct only that level; however, since my spine was unstable, that was out of the question. I would need more comprehensive procedures to finally correct my curved spine. This would be a life-altering surgery that would take many hours and require an intensive recovery over many months.

My physical therapist, Megan Cullen, and I worked hard to reduce pain and stay strong leading up to the surgery. We wanted my body to be as strong as possible to prepare it for its biggest challenge yet. She walked me through so many dimensions of the surgery and my life after it. We talked about my quality of life, which had dwindled as my pain progressed over the years: I canceled plans or didn't make any. I traveled for work when I had to, but I would work from my bed with my laptop anytime I was home. I lived on Tylenol, ice packs, my heating pad, and my TENS unit. I got into the water as much as possible even though I could no longer kick my legs to swim. I wore buoyancy shorts to help keep my hips up when I swam, powering through the water only using my upper body. By discussing these issues with Megan, I was able to see the potential for this major surgery—I had made so many concessions to scoliosis over such a long period of time that I could not always see how much it had derailed my hopes and dreams for life. I began to look forward to the procedure and the life that awaited me after it.

On October 30, 2018, I had two surgeries: an anterior approach to place interbody cages at L4/5 and L5/S1 and a second surgery called an XLIF, where Dr. Tantorski went in through my ribs and replaced my diseased discs with shiny new prosthetic discs for my remaining lumber vertebrae. Two days later, he went in through my back to straighten my spine. My spine had been in a curved position for most of my life. With rods, hooks, and screws, he straightened my spine and fused it from T10 to S1.

I woke up from my final surgery to my sister brushing my hair and to more pain than I could have fathomed. The searing pain in my ribs was unexpected; it hadn't occurred to me that I would have this related to the XLIF part of my surgery. I was in the hospital for about a week, and it was a blur of vital signs, pain medication, physical therapy, and doctors coming in and out of my room. I was so grateful for my family, the amazing hospital staff, and the wonderful care I received. I did advocate for Boost in the hospital to rebuild my strength—I could not eat much due to nausea and lack of appetite. I told hospital staff that I could not recover on half a grilled cheese sandwich per day and that my doctor would order supplements for me, which he did.

Life After Major Spinal Surgery

Following my 2018 surgery, I had a long road ahead of me both physically and emotionally. I faced many challenges as I spent months recovering. I was on disability for three months, and once I was cleared to work, I still needed to work from home as I was unable to drive. My full-time job was, and still is, remote with travel. I was isolated at home and in a toxic long-term relationship, so being at home more was not good for me.

After this surgery, my body was not my own; it was different now. Although I hated my "rib hump," it had been a part of me, and it was no longer there. I now had three large scars, over two feet in length, and the one on my stomach bothered me the most. It did not heal well, requiring numerous treatments for keloids and pain. These treatments made the appearance of the scar worse, and I could not bear to look at myself in the mirror.

At about five months post-op, I started to experience mood swings: I was angry and would feel panic in the middle of the night. My heart would race for no reason, and I struggled to keep my thoughts from running away from me. I couldn't understand what was wrong with me. Then, it occurred to me: *This feels very familiar.* I was experiencing symptoms of PTSD. Because of my clinical training and prior life experiences, I knew I needed to seek help from others.

I received so much support from my physical therapist, Megan. She helped me recover and learn how not to walk like a robot, and she was there for my emotional struggles. On many days, the mental hurdle was much greater than the physical one. She would push me physically while also being a soft landing for my emotions and validating my feelings.

I briefly saw a psychologist at that rehab hospital, but she did not understand body image disturbance and invalidated my experience, so after two sessions, I did not return. She tried to make me feel better by telling me that I looked like a fitness model, and I explained to her that my body image wasn't distorted and that I didn't think I was unattractive—I just was uncomfortable in this new body with my hips and ribs in a new place and new scars.

My surgery gave me a new life and the courage to do so many things. It gave me the strength to end a relationship that I had been in for almost a decade that was toxic and abusive. Before my surgery, I felt unlovable due to my limitations, pain, and body image related to my disability. After surgery, I still had pain, limitations, and more scars, but I had the chance at a new life, and that meant all of my life, not just parts.

Final Thoughts

My life has changed so much in the years that followed my surgeries. I now do obstacle course races with a stellar group of people who have become close friends. I continue to thrive in the eating disorder field and do what I can to help in whatever capacity I can, whether that is by being a group leader, chapter president, mentor, or friend. I still have some limits, but my life is far greater than I could have ever imagined.

As I look back at photos of the years before and after surgery, I feel a wide range of emotions. In the past, I learned to put on a pretty smile and act as if everything was okay. Over time, I learned to be honest when others asked how I was feeling. "Yes, I am in pain today." "No I didn't sleep much." "Yes I'm frustrated with my body." "Ugh, I don't want to recover from another thing." That openness and authenticity has changed my relationships and allowed me to honor myself. I get to choose if I want to show up or stay home and rest—that embodiment has been another skill I have learned over time.

Part 2

Definitions

To begin to understand how chronic illness and eating disorders overlap and to treat them together, it is vital to explore the terms and concepts that accompany these conditions. This section of the book defines chronic medical conditions, chronic pain, and pain psychology, along with their relationships to eating disorders. I also identify common comorbid medical conditions and eating disorders.

In Part 2, I start by discussing how to assess eating disorders in individuals with chronic health conditions. Additionally, I will review the different types of pain as well as concepts such as pain tolerance and pain threshold. This section will explore mental defeat and chronic pain as risk factors for suicide, and I will examine body image issues related to chronic illness, including recommendations for assessment.

Each chapter will include relevant research findings and conclude with practical suggestions for clinicians. I will also share pertinent social media posts from my Instagram account, which I use to document my journey after life-altering back surgery in 2018.

- Chapter 2: What Is a Chronic Medical Condition and How Does It Relate to an Eating Disorder?
- Chapter 3: Chronic Pain and Pain Psychology
- Chapter 4: The Intersection of Body Image and Chronic Illness

DOI: 10.4324/9781003500254-3

Chapter 2

What Is a Chronic Medical Condition and How Does It Relate to an Eating Disorder?

To begin the journey of understanding chronic illnesses and disordered eating, I want to define chronic illness and how it intersects with potential disordered eating. Chronic illnesses are not all the same, but often they are invisible to the wider world while being completely consuming and agonizing to a person living with one or even more of them. Understanding how chronic illness impacts people's lives will better illuminate any eating disorders they may experience. I will offer some exercises and tips for clinicians in working with clients with chronic illnesses and eating disorders at the end of the chapter.

What Is a Chronic Illness?

A disease is considered *chronic* when it is not curable but has no mortal outcome. It can last a very long time and is usually progressive with alternating periods of illness and wellness. Some people with chronic illnesses are born with a genetic condition, while others may be diagnosed later in life.

Living with a chronic illness requires flexibility, adaptation, and compassion. The chronically ill person repeatedly experiences feelings of grief—at the beginning of their diagnosis, with the progression of the disease, and with each setback. Chronic illnesses can vacillate unexpectedly, making it difficult for a person to predict their day-to-day lives. For me, this often shows up in my ability to be active and fully participate in my job, including work travel. Another example in my life is how I move my body for exercise. I am currently in a period of life where I cannot run. However, to stay active, I was able to come up with an adaptive way to swim where I don't have to rotate my head. It's my own style. Over time, my abilities continue to change. My adaptations and changes may not be recognized or understood by others, and this is how many people with chronic illness navigate their lives.

DOI: 10.4324/9781003500254-4

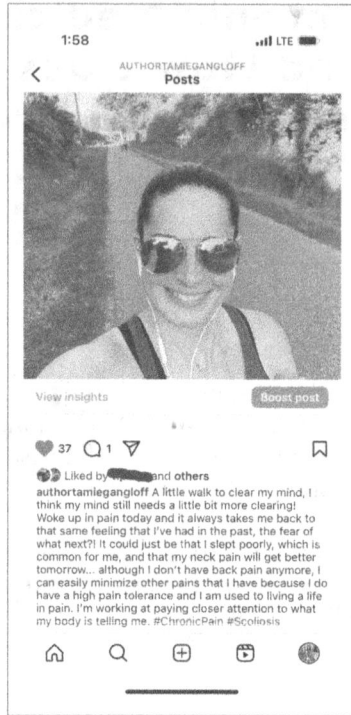

Clearing My Head

The Physical, Mental, and Emotional Challenges of Chronic Illness

Chronic disease causes a disruption of self, both physically and socially. It becomes challenging to separate the person from the illness. I know this firsthand. Scoliosis is a part of who I am, but it isn't my entirety. Most people who meet me will find out that I have scoliosis, and the more we talk, they will learn about how it has changed my life and also made me who I am. It has caused a great deal of distress and also instilled a level of resilience in me that is almost unshakable. Sometimes my confidence is shaken, but I am typically able to work towards finding a solution and get stronger physically and emotionally. I imagine that most people living with chronic illnesses would tell a similar story. Living with a chronic condition disrupts a person's life, but they have to continue to live, even if that is much different from the way others around them do. This can be an opportunity for someone with a chronic illness to persevere, but it can also be exhausting physically, emotionally, and spiritually. It may even trigger other factors in someone's life, such as an eating disorder.

Stress Associated with Chronic Illness

Stress comes from the chronic illness for a variety of reasons, including limitations in daily life, the physical pain often accompanying it, and the tension it creates in relationships, socializing, family, and career.

Chronic pain and illness can be debilitating and intolerable, and there can be a significant loss of quality of life. The loss of quality of life often is one of the greatest causes of distress and depression in those living with chronic illnesses. It often shows up as a part of an injury or illness; however, it is its own diagnosis and condition (Mills, 2019).

Someone living with a chronic illness may experience anxiety, uncertainty, and grief about a future that may have additional limits and challenges due to the illness. This fear can be crippling at times and result in a diminished sense of self.

Reframing Chronic Illness with Clients

To begin to treat someone experiencing an eating disorder and living with a chronic illness, it may be useful to help them reframe their situation. This work might begin with reframing the chronic illness. In a search for synonyms for *chronic*, I attempted to find a more positive word, or just a different one. I didn't find words that I liked, and many had a negative connotation, such as persistent, serial, stubborn, incorrigible, and ceaseless. However, I jumped on a few others. The terms that felt somewhat positive were *long-term* and *steady*. Thinking about a chronic illness with these more optimistic synonyms can help someone rethink their condition to help them have a more positive outlook on life. Both long-term and steady imply a *relationship* with the condition. Being "in a relationship" with something implies that a person can work on, grow from, and have a positive connection with the condition. It might sound silly to a client to suggest this metaphor, but encourage them to give it a try. This can be the first step in changing the narrative of living with a chronic illness. After all, the relationship we have with ourselves is the most significant one throughout our lifespan. *See Exercise 2.1 later in this chapter for instructions on leading this exercise with your clients.*

Let me frame this concept around my own life to give you a more concrete example of how to do this with a client: *I have a long-term relationship with my scoliosis; I am going steady with my titanium!* Does this sound silly? Absolutely. I reread that last sentence and laughed out loud. Sometimes we have to laugh at ourselves. So let's keep going with this: *This is the longest relationship I have had and will have—we will be together for the rest of my life.* I can choose to embrace it as part of who I am, and, as with any relationship, there will be good times and bad ... in sickness and in health!

In eating disorder treatment, we often discuss the eating disorder and healthy self and the creation of a dialogue between them. This reinforces the relationship between them as partners, integrating them together. We don't need to "get rid of" the eating disorder voice – it is a part of us, and we need to listen to what it has to say. As we learn to have a dialogue, it can help clients recover.

Some theories work on getting rid of the eating disorder self; however, I trained under Carolyn Costin whose philosophy is not to make an enemy of the eating disorder self but to learn from it and strengthen the person's healthy self to take over its job. With this work, we don't get rid of the eating disorder part of self; we get rid of the destructive behaviors it uses by strengthening the healthy self and getting it back in charge. The goal is integration, so the person no longer has two parts but becomes whole. Key 2 in *8 Keys to Recovery from an Eating Disorder* focuses on this specifically. Through treatment, "what used to be an eating disorder self becomes a part of your healthy self that serves as an alert system that something needs to be attended to" (Costin & Schubert Grabb, 2011).

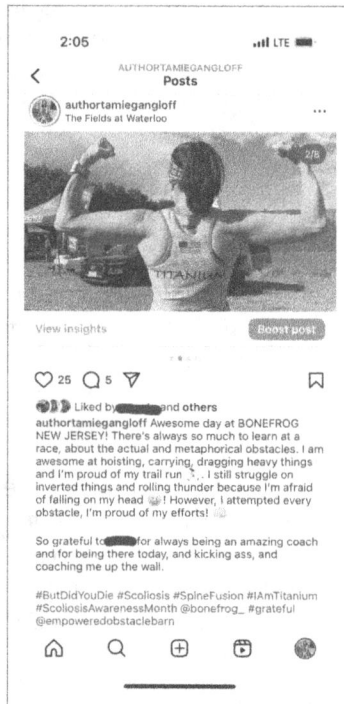

Titanium

In my case, I applied this concept by accepting that my chronic illness was a part of me, and I nicknamed it "Titanium." I learned from it and began to see how it was a part of me that could be incredibly strong. Many parts of my body are titanium after my life-altering surgery in 2018. During this procedure, my spine had a makeover with rods, screws, hooks, and prosthetic discs and now has a lot of metal, including titanium. Although I still have scoliosis and its complications, my titanium gave me my life back. I accept this part of my self, listen to it but put my healthy self in charge of responding.

Intersection of Disordered Eating and Chronic Illness

While chronic illnesses do not inherently connect with disordered eating, the two can be linked. There are many medical conditions that overlap with eating disorders. The illness may predispose someone to an eating disorder, as the eating disorder may cause them to have a limited diet and may contribute to the development of an eating disorder. Other times, the illness isn't especially causative, but it makes disordered eating and illness more complicated to treat. Oftentimes, chronic illness makes eating disorder recovery more complex because diet and exercise often play a role in the treatment of the chronic condition.

Unfortunately, eating disorder inventories and assessments are not tailored to those with chronic illness, making it difficult for us to assess an accurate percentage of those with eating disorders and a chronic medical condition. However, the lack of data should not prevent clinicians from connecting them when evaluating, treating, and understanding clients. Furthermore, this is a topic that needs more research and should be studied by those within the fields of chronic illness, eating disorders, and nutrition. I will highlight some of my own data on the intersection between chronic illness and disordered eating throughout the book (and my first-person narrative in this book directly shows how the two conditions can impact one's life). I welcome others to take up research on this topic as well.

Diet-Related Chronic Health Conditions

Diet-related chronic health conditions include but are not limited to celiac disease, irritable bowel disease, Crohn's, cystic fibrosis, and type 1 diabetes. These medical conditions require patients to follow a regulated plan for eating, food restrictions, and close monitoring, causing them to overfocus on food and their body, out of necessity. These food restrictions may lead them to feel different from their peers, and that can lead to isolation or depressive symptoms. These concerns, coupled with other risk factors, including social media, trauma, and a family history of disordered eating, may lead to an eating disorder. It is important for medical providers to pay close attention to the children and adolescents with these chronic illnesses and monitor them not only for depression and anxiety but also for eating disorders as well.

While digestive-related chronic illnesses can predispose someone to disordered eating, any chronic illness can intersect with an eating disorder. Oftentimes, it is the perfect storm, along with other precipitating factors, that can contribute to the development of an eating disorder.

I will highlight two chronic illnesses and frame how they may contribute to an eating disorder. These examples are not exhaustive but are merely an analysis of how a chronic illness and eating disorder may manifest in someone.

Type 1 Diabetes and Eating Disorders

Type 1 diabetes is a chronic condition without a cure. Receiving this diagnosis is life-altering and is often diagnosed after a period of illness in which someone has lost a significant amount of weight. Adapting to a new life of insulin dependence and counting carbs can be very stressful for the patient and family. Research shows that the prevalence of eating disorders is higher in those with type 1 diabetes than in the general population. The child and adolescent population may be particularly vulnerable to the development of an eating disorder following a type 1 diabetes diagnosis because the illness's symptoms and focus on food following diagnosis, without having the maturity or information available on how to manage the condition healthily. Those with type 1 diabetes may withhold insulin for weight loss purposes. A recent study reported that 42% of those diagnosed with an eating disorder and type 1 diabetes have withheld insulin for weight loss purposes (Quick et al., 2013). Although not a formal diagnosis, diabulimia can be a very dangerous disorder and requires a high level of medical oversight to treat correctly.

Cystic Fibrosis and Eating Disorders

Cystic fibrosis (CF) causes damage to the lungs and digestive system. CF affects the cells that produce mucus and causes it to become thick. As it relates to digestion, the mucus blocks the tubes that carry digestive enzymes, so nutrients are not absorbed. Due to the inability to absorb nutrients, it is often difficult for a CF patient to maintain a normal body weight (Mayo Clinic, 2024). Treatment includes vitamin and mineral supplements, digestive enzymes, and a higher fat percentage in diet, and, at times, feeding tubes may become necessary. This can create eating-related issues, as someone living with CF may not understand how to maintain a healthy weight while living with their illness. An eating disorder clinician or medical provider can work with a client to make sure they understand the impact of their illness on their diet and body image, and help them overcome any challenges they may encounter.

Similar Tracks for Understanding Chronic Illnesses and Eating Disorders

In eating disorder recovery, we often talk of bringing the dark into the light. The eating-disordered part of us may come from a dark place; it may have developed out of necessity to protect us from harm or trauma and/or from a place of necessity and strength. These sources of the eating disorder may have many qualities that, when brought into the light, can become our greatest assets.

The same is true for those of us with a chronic medical condition. Our perceived weaknesses and struggles may lead us to our inner strength and resolve. Sports injury psychology calls this *sports injury-related growth*, and we see something very similar in chronic conditions. It is also often called *posttraumatic growth*; the terms can be interchangeable. There is personal growth that comes from every hardship a person living with a chronic illness encounters, whether that is surgery, a flare, or another setback. The recovery from those times can be times of growth. This growth also allows us to deepen our sense of self as a whole person instead of our list of diagnoses.

Growth from struggle is also true for eating disorders; they are often characterized by a loss of sense of self, and recovery requires intensive work to gain that sense of self. When someone has both a chronic illness and an eating disorder, that work is exponentially more challenging. If one's identity consists of a list of diagnoses, it is often difficult to identify who they are aside from that list, whether it is mental health or medical.

Recognizing the Presence of Chronic Illness when Treating Eating Disorders

In 2024, I began my presentation at the International Association for Eating Disorder Professionals Symposium in Orlando, Florida, with the following two questions:

1 Does anyone here identify as having a chronic illness?
2 Do you have a client that has a chronic illness?

Many clinicians did not know that they had a chronic illness until they heard it defined during my presentation. Numerous clinicians raised their hands, and some reached out later that day and in the following days and months regarding their own health.

As clinicians, we are called on to do our own work on ourselves. Have you been living with a chronic condition? You might find that your chronic condition has impacted your life in many ways. You may be able to understand your condition and your clients better by recognizing your own limitations brought on by chronic illness and the many ways a chronic illness must be managed and understood. This recognition will not only help your clinical practice, but it may also give you the opportunity to better understand yourself. If you do have a chronic illness, I hope you can take the time you need to make sure you take care of yourself. Consider my story within these pages and the many lessons I have learned that have improved not only my quality of life but also my work with clients and in the professional field. Remember that there are many opportunities for personal growth when we come to terms with our own challenges.

When I asked the second question about having clients with chronic illnesses, almost every hand went up. While this was unsurprising, considering the prevalence of chronic illnesses among the general population, some of the feedback that I received showed the disconnect in how clinicians work with these clients. The feedback from one of my friends, a certified eating disorder dietitian, was that she was nervous to take on such a client, as she didn't know much about their illness and did not want to say the wrong thing. Another therapist asked how she could help if she did not have her own lived experience with that illness. These comments raise the imperative for more research to be done in this intersection, and the exercises that follow suggest ways a clinician can begin to recognize and appropriately treat someone with disordered eating and a chronic illness.

Remember this as a clinician: We know that although it can be helpful to have shared lived experiences, it is not necessary to share those experiences to help others. Many get into our field due to our own recovery; however, I know many phenomenal clinicians who came to love this work but who do not have their own personal lived experience with an eating disorder.

Suggestions for Treating the Disordered Eating Client with a Chronic Illness

Be Curious

My first piece of advice here is to *be curious*. In my own situation, scoliosis impacts 1 in 40 people, so I have a good chance of meeting someone with my condition. However, many conditions are much rarer. You do not need to have the answers regarding diagnosis, prognosis, and medical symptoms for someone's chronic illness. *As clinicians, our responsibility is to gain an understanding of our clients, their experiences, and their struggles, and come from a place of compassion and empathy to help them live their lives beyond their eating disorder and medical condition.*

We are here to join with our clients, which means that we do not need to have all of the answers about them but be open to them discussing their health condition. If you open the door, they will tell you all about their illness. Those with a chronic illness often learn to minimize symptoms so they don't worry friends and family. Clients may feel like a burden on their loved ones, so it may feel like a relief to respond to your curiosity without worrying that you might fall apart.

You are here to guide a client through living life with their illness and all of the implications of that. Once you learn more about your client and their illness, I suggest you do your own research to learn more about it. After you do your research, bring that into your sessions—your client will feel seen, heard, and cared for in this action. Ask more questions. This will let them know that you are invested in them, and they will feel that you are in it with them. *Keep in mind that just as every eating disorder presents differently, so does every medical condition.* You will then have the opportunity to examine the intersection of their medical condition and eating disorder.

I would recommend following the advice from one of my mentors, Carolyn Costin, when it comes to someone with an eating disorder and a chronic illness:

1 Show up
2 Pay attention
3 Tell the truth without judgment
4 Don't be attached to the results

This framework will keep you curious as you work with clients and allow them to bring all their cards to the table, which should help with eating disorder recovery.

Try This Exercise to Help Your Client Frame Their Chronic Illness

Earlier in this chapter, I described an exercise for someone with a chronic illness to use to reframe their condition into something they are *in relationship with* versus *sentenced to deal with*, or some other negative connection. While you may not understand all aspects of a client's chronic health condition, walking through this exercise may help you relate to them better and give them a more positive outlook on their condition. This exercise could help open your client up as you work with them on their eating disorder.

Exercise 2.1: Build a Relationship With Your Chronic Illness

What name would you give your chronic illness? Let's be creative and choose something fun.

Many with eating disorders choose to use the acronym ED to externalize their eating disorder. Your illness name can be an acronym or something that has special meaning for you.

Name of your illness(es): _____

Nickname(s): _____

Next, think about how you can be in a relationship with your chronic illness. It might help to think of your closest friendships, the friends who are there no matter what. I have some friendships that have endured through many years of challenges, yet they remain in my circle. Those strong friendships can survive difficult conversations and life challenges and strengthen as a result. If you do not have a friendship like this in your life, that is okay! It might help to think of others in your life that you see these qualities in.

Since you will be in a relationship with your condition, think about the ways you would relate to it. Qualities of relationships include:

- Trust
- Affirmation
- Healthy boundaries
- Nurturing
- Kindness and support
- Acceptance
- Non-judgment
- Grace
- Forgiveness
- Communication
- Empathy

Try to use these attributes in your relationship with your illness. It can be easy to feel frustrated and defeated with yourself, but reframing your chronic illness as a lifelong relationship could be helpful. This dialogue and reframe works with the eating disorder/healthy self as well!

You may use negative words when you experience setbacks from your chronic illness like: *I am so frustrated with my body, I am tired of being in pain, feeling exhausted, I just want to have one good day!*

Here's an example of how you could talk to your illness instead by using the nickname you assigned it. Remember to talk to it as you would speak to a dear friend (in this example, I use the nickname for my illness, Titanium): *I am frustrated with Titanium today! I know that she is doing the best she can, and I am trusting that she is doing everything she can to care for us.*

Understand a Client's Lived Experiences

Another way you can show support to your client about their chronic illness is to understand their lived experience. To navigate the conversation about a client's chronic illness, consider these statements and questions I have heard during groups for clients with eating disorders and chronic illnesses:

- How do I validate my needs and experience when they are misunderstood?
- How do I validate myself?
- How long until there is a flare, new injury, or new degeneration?
- Will I be able to get the treatment that I need with my medical condition *and* my eating disorder?
- This is *not* a choice – neither my eating disorder nor my illness is my choice.
- My chronic illness can be "made less difficult by taking care of myself."
- It is easy to gaslight myself—"I can't recover from my eating disorder because I have this illness."
- When will the other shoe drop?
- I have lost faith … in myself and in my recovery.
- How long until I lose something else?
- Comparison: I'm not disabled enough. My disability is invisible.
- I feel like I have to justify my needs to take care of myself.
- I have to advocate for myself on all fronts of my care.

Summary

A chronic illness can be congenital or developed later in life, and it is chronic when it lasts for more than one year. While we know that there is an intersection between chronic illness and eating disorders, research in this area is lacking. Diet-related chronic health conditions may have a higher incidence of disordered eating than other chronic health conditions. The emotional and mental impact of the illness is significant. The disruption of self that is caused by the chronic illness may lead to mental health struggles including eating disorders. The use of narrative therapy to rename the illness may help to allow it to become a part of a client's view of self instead of who they are.

In the next chapter, we will examine chronic pain and pain psychology.

References

Costin, C., & Gwen Schubert Grabb. (2011). *8 Keys to Recovery from an Eating Disorder: Effective Strategies from Therapeutic Practice and Personal Experience (8 Keys to Mental Health)*. W. W. Norton & Company. https://doi.org/10.3945/an.112.003608

Mayo Clinic. (2024). *Cystic fibrosis*. www.mayoclinic.org/diseases-conditions/cystic-fibrosis/symptoms-causes/syc-20353700

Mills, S. E. E., Nicolson, K. P., & Smith, B. H. (2019). Chronic pain: A review of its epidemiology and associated factors in population-based Studies. *British Journal of Anaesthesia*, *123*(2), e273–e283. https://doi.org/10.1016/j.bja.2019.03.023

Quick, V. M., Byrd-Bredbenner, C., & Neumark-Sztainer, D. (2013). Chronic illness and disordered eating: A discussion of the literature. *Advances in Nutrition*, *4*(3), 277–286.

Chapter 3

Chronic Pain and Pain Psychology

Many people with a chronic illness will experience chronic pain. This is pain that lasts a long time and may flare if triggered. Clinicians should try to understand any chronic pain their clients experience as they treat them for disordered eating. It is important to have a complete understanding of how chronic pain impacts a client's daily life and behaviors because it can actually work in tandem with pain experienced with an eating disorder. It is imperative that a clinician is aware of a client's mental well-being during eating disorder treatment and conscious of how chronic illness may contribute to it. This chapter will address chronic pain and offer ways for a clinician to evaluate chronic pain with their clients.

Chronic Pain Defined

Chronic pain is defined as pain that lasts for more than three months; it can be consistent or may come and go (Cleveland Clinic, 2024). Chronic pain is one of the primary reasons people seek medical attention. Our bodies are sensitive, and pain is a signal that there is something wrong that needs to be tended to. *Pain is communicated between your nerves, spinal cord, and brain.* However, if these signals have been firing for many years, it becomes too much to endure. Many people with chronic illnesses have lived with pain for most of their lives. Personally, although I was diagnosed with scoliosis as a kid, my chronic pain did not start until my mid-twenties. However, now that I am middle-aged, this means I have lived with it for over half of my life.

Someone with chronic pain may be hypervigilant and is always waiting for the other shoe to drop. *An important goal for someone with a chronic illness is the ability to acknowledge the pain while pursuing valued life activities in the presence of pain.*

DOI: 10.4324/9781003500254-5

Types of Pain

There are several types of pain (Santos-Longhurst, 2018), and someone with a chronic illness may experience one or more of them.

- Acute—usually sharp pain with a known cause; it is short-lived and is caused by an accident, injury, surgery, or broken bones.
- Musculoskeletal—pain associated with bones, tendons, joints, ligaments, and muscle. This can be due to an injury or a disability.
- Neuropathic—also known as nerve pain. This type of pain may be caused by nerve impingement or by a disease such as diabetes or shingles.
- Visceral—results from injuries to your internal organs.
- Inflammatory—this pain is in response to an injury or disease that causes an inflammatory response. Autoimmune disorders such as lupus or rheumatoid arthritis cause inflammatory pain.

But How Does It Really Feel?

Pain is *subjective*, meaning that two people with the same diagnosis, injury, illness, or surgery can experience pain in different ways with varying levels of pain, pain threshold, and ability to tolerate the pain. Sharp, burning, stabbing, dull, pressure, cramping, crippling, stiff are just a few descriptors often used to describe pain.

On December 27, 2022, I had a personal training session and an encouraging appointment with a doctor that advised a transforaminal steroid injection at the T9 level, and I got approval from Dr. T. While the procedure may not happen until February, I'm grateful for the chance to find relief and continue my wellness journey.

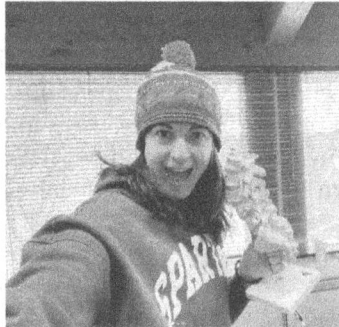

A Day in the Life of a Chronic Spine Patient

Pain Threshold and Pain Tolerance

Your *pain threshold* is the point at which a sensation becomes painful. It's not the same thing as tolerance, which is how much you can handle (Torres, 2022). We see examples of this in people with a high threshold for heat or cold as well as noise. If you have been exposed to temperature extremes or loud sounds for a long period of time, the threshold at which these things become bothersome is much lower. *Pain threshold also tends to lower as we age.*

Pain tolerance is our ability to tolerate pain and is different for everyone based on biological factors, experience, trauma, and mental health challenges. Prolonged exposure to pain can increase pain tolerance, and people develop the ability to endure more pain. This can be helpful in someone with a chronic pain condition; however, we then learn to ignore our body's signals. Much like we unlearn our hunger and fullness signals, when we ignore them for a long period of time, a similar phenomenon occurs when we tolerate pain for long periods of time.

Can It Be Dangerous to Have a High Pain Tolerance?

Absolutely. My ability to endure pain is significant. I have pain in many different parts of my body on a regular basis and some areas are more sensitive than others. Out of the necessity of life, I have learned to manage my pain and also sometimes I have to ignore it to get through the day. The ability to compartmentalize life can be useful. For example, if you just had an argument with your spouse, you might need to compartmentalize it if you have to go into an important work meeting. The ability to contain that situation and those emotions is necessary to focus and be present in the moment to do your work. The same is true for pain. I do not recommend that someone hide or ignore their pain, and I am also acknowledging that it happens out of necessity.

In a recent social media post, I talked about smiling and *looking pretty for the pictures*. I have a job that I love, and it is public-facing. You will see an example of this in the next chapter. This means that no matter what my pain level is on any given day, I show up and present, drive far to a meeting, host events, and carry out the most important part of my job: talking to clients and families. If I am hurting, my ability to do those things can be diminished. I often have to psych myself up to show up with a smile. Sometimes, I am fully engaged and present and, other times, I *smile pretty for the pictures*, meaning that I show up and give it all I have in the presence of pain.

The ability to tolerate and endure may be born out of necessity; however, it can be dangerous. If I can compartmentalize my pain or ignore my pain, I am missing out on very important signals. For example, I did not know that I had a fractured clavicle until six weeks later, and I did not realize that my big toe was broken at the joint! I have become more hypervigilant about pain as I now understand that by the time I am sensing pain and it is not tolerable, my body has been sending the signals for a while and my pain or injury can be much worse than I realize. This is where I rely on my patient, kind, and compassionate medical team.

Why Is It Dangerous for Someone with an Eating Disorder to Have a High Pain Tolerance?

Simply stated, many eating disorder symptoms cause pain, whether it is purging, laxative abuse, overexercise, the pain of a binge, or the burning sensation of restriction. *An eating disorder is physically painful.* As someone suffers with an eating disorder, their ability to ignore their body's cues for hunger, fullness, and pain increases. Sometimes, they crave that pain as a form of self-harm or a distraction from the emotionally painful issues in their lives.

With what we know about pain threshold and pain tolerance in the chronically ill patient, when we add an eating disorder into the mix, we typically have a person that has a very high pain threshold and tolerance. *This becomes dangerous because not only may they be hiding their symptom use, but they are not fully feeling the pain associated with it.* If their body is sending distress signals, they are not feeling the intensity of them, and it may be too late by the time they sense that something is wrong. As we work on reconnecting to the body's signals, we need to do this for all cues, including pain. We may not change someone's threshold or tolerance for pain, but we can bring awareness to it so they know that they might need to seek medical advice or take care of themselves in this way. Many people with chronic illnesses and eating disorders have learned to push through the pain and need to learn how to live their lives and acknowledge their pain to heal from an eating disorder and better manage chronic illness.

Chronic Pain as a Risk Factor for Suicide

The *Journal of Pain Research* states that "a U.S. study found that 8.8% of suicide deaths involved chronic pain. Over half of those individuals noted pain as a factor in their suicide notes" (Themelis et al., 2023, p.11). The mental defeat of living with chronic pain can lead to suicidal thinking. We know that many factors are at play when someone becomes suicidal; however, this is a significant factor in the chronic illness community. In a 2023 study, Themelis et al. discovered: "Awareness of the prospective links from mental defeat, depression, perceived stress, head pain, and active smoking status to increased suicide risk in patients with chronic pain may offer a novel avenue for assessment and preventative intervention" (Themelis, 2023, p.11).

Mental Defeat

Mental defeat is noted as being more causative of suicidality than anxiety, depression, or catastrophic thinking. Those of us with chronic pain have all felt fear of the future and sometimes cannot fathom getting through another day at this pain level. Fear of the future and loss of quality of life are contributing factors to mental defeat. Feelings that it will never get better lead to this level of hopelessness. Compounding this is the anxiety surrounding the pain; this anxiety can also serve to increase the amount of pain someone is in. Stress lowers the threshold for pain, actually increasing pain levels (PainScale, n.d.). Anxiety leads to increased pain levels, thus causing people to become more anxious because they are in more pain. The fear of the pain creates a vicious cycle. Personally, my tolerance for pain decreases because of the fear surrounding what this means for my life, how it is impacting it today, and anticipation of when it will get worse.

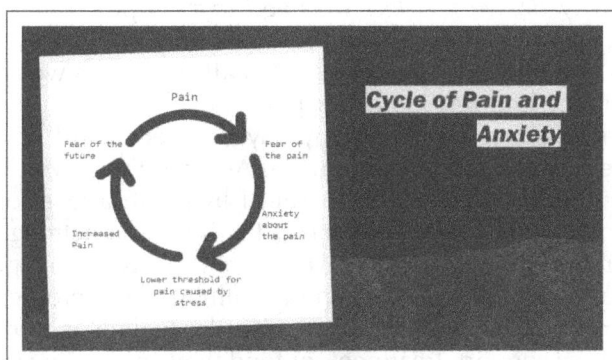

Rating Pain and Avoiding Comparisons to Others' Pain

When sharing with someone, whether it is in group or on an Instagram reel, I never rate my pain with a number. Numbers, in general, promote comparison and can bring anxiety. Comparison is not helpful at all and if someone hears a specific pain number, they can fall into a "not sick enough" mindset.

If no one asks about my pain and limitations, I don't typically offer the information unless I feel like I have to. The "have to" can be because I have to say no to something or because I need help. I also find myself explaining that "It's okay, it's just my normal" to make others feel comfortable with it. Studies show that pain and empathy are linked and that it is human nature to not want to see others in pain. As a result, many of us have learned to hide or minimize our physical and emotional pain so that we don't make others feel uncomfortable. The experience is similar for someone with an eating disorder. Someone with an eating disorder may go to great lengths to hide their struggle, whether that is hiding symptom use or wearing clothing to hide a changing body. When asked about their struggles, they may minimize how they are feeling and the significance of their current struggles, whether that is symptom use or their comorbid anxiety or depression.

I have had people tell me they shouldn't complain about their bad back because mine is so much worse. My response usually is that I am used to it, and it is my normal, so my struggle might not be as significant as theirs. *When we compare, there almost always is a judgment attached to it.* It is human nature to struggle with being objective. If we could be 100% objective and self-reflective, we wouldn't need therapy or friends!

When I had a conversation with my friend Agamemnon (you will meet Agamemnon and Zephyr in Chapter 15), he posed an important question: *Why do we feel like we need to earn pain relief?* My other friend, Zephyr, and I talked about how we only will take something if the pain is bad enough. "Bad enough" is all relative as we all have different tolerance and thresholds for pain. I expressed that I would take Tylenol if my pain is impacting my day or sleep, and I will even use a lidocaine patch if my pain is severe. As I see those words, I know I am not being fully honest with myself. I live with a level of pain that is my normal. A truer statement is that I will take something if my pain is significantly above my normal level of pain. I have a feeling that this is accurate for many people with chronic illness and chronic pain. This is similar to someone with an eating disorder feeling as if they have to earn emotional support, treatment, or food they enjoy. They may feel the need to be sick enough to earn the support of their loved ones or receive eating disorder care.

Treating Pain

Everyone does different things to manage their pain. Some will use CBD, THC, and other pain medications. This is not the forum for that; however, I want to acknowledge that we all need to do what works to manage our own pain. Personally, I choose not to try CBD or THC as there is the potential that it could impact my sobriety. That being said, using a medication or supplement of any kind is personal and is a decision for you to make with your medical providers and treatment team.

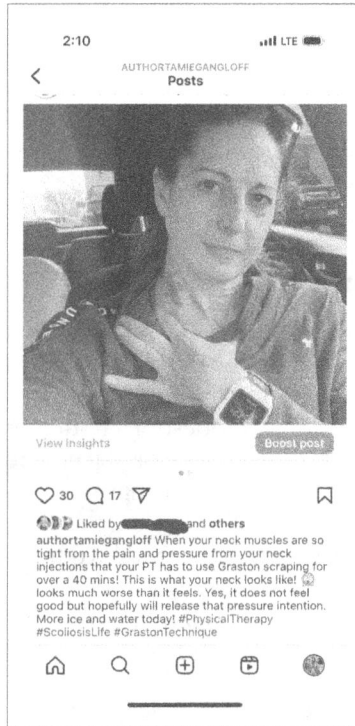

Treating Pain in a Variety of Ways

Tips for a Client with Chronic Illness: Plan for a Pain Flare

This is something I learned from my favorite sports medicine doctor, Dr. Payne (yes, that's her real name!). We talk about planning for pain flare. We aren't hoping that we won't have any pain; we are assuming that we will have a flare and we are planning for it. When we plan ahead for this and know that it will happen, it lessens the amount of anxiety and panic. When I have pain, I know my plan and I put it into action. This doesn't mean that I will not be upset that it is happening; however, I won't have to guess about what to do next. Similar to having a plan for riding the wave of an urge to use eating disorder symptoms. When the intensity of the urge is high, you might not be able to think through what you need to do to help, but when you work on a plan and know what helps ahead of time, you can access it when you need it.

My pain flare plan includes heat, ice, cryotherapy, lidocaine patches, over-the-counter pain relievers, gentle movement, TENS unit, and reaching out to my medical team. I also reach out to my friends that can relate and offer support. I need a combination of mental and physical support.

Suggestions and Activities for Clinicians

When meeting with our clients, we always need to assess pain levels and suicidality. When a dietitian meets with their eating disorder client, they are reviewing meal plans, symptom use, hunger, and fullness cues. Oftentimes, unless we ask the specific questions—such as "Did you purge?" or "Have you had urges to overexercise?" or "Have you been restricting your snacks?"—clients often don't volunteer that information. Typically, clients find it challenging to flat-out lie when asked the specifics. We need to treat pain and suicidal assessment the same way we treat questions about meal plans and eating disorder symptom urges and use.

Clients with eating disorders have an increased risk of suicide, and coupled with chronic illness and pain, that risk is elevated.

Exercise 3.1: Use the Suicide Risk Screening Tool

I recommend using the Suicide Risk Screening Tool by the National Institute of Mental Health (2024). Simply asking if someone has had suicidal thinking is not comprehensive enough. This questionnaire is comprehensive and specific.

1   In the past few weeks, have you wished you were dead?
2   In the past few weeks, have you felt that your family would be better off if you were dead?
3   In the past week, have you had thoughts about killing yourself? (If yes, how? When?)
4   Have you ever tried to kill yourself?

If patients said yes to any of these questions, ask them if they are having thoughts of killing themselves now.

Exercise 3.2: Address a Client's Pain

This might feel uncomfortable as we typically don't ask these questions in a therapy setting. Questions about pain are often asked by a physical therapist or in another medical setting. However, aren't we always assessing pain levels? We check in with our clients about their level of emotional distress, so this is no different.

There are many pain scales that you can use. We have all seen the posters of the faces rating pain on a 1–10 scale. As I mentioned earlier in this chapter, it is relative and we all rate pain differently. The number isn't the most important part—what that number means to that client is most important. If your client typically rates their pain at a three, but it has been a five or more for the past few weeks, that is cause for concern as they are likely experiencing emotional distress as a result.

Examples of questions to as a client:

1 Rate your pain on a scale of 1–10.
2 Describe your pain (burning, stabbing, aching, etc.).
3 Does your pain keep you awake at night?

   a How much sleep are you getting at night?
   b Do you feel rested when you get up in the morning?

4 Is this a new pain?
5 If so, are you aware of what triggered this pain (new injury, pain flare, etc.)?
6 Does anything lessen the pain (ice, heat, medication, rest, etc.)?
7 When did your pain start?
8 How do you feel about the pain (anxious, sad, frustrated, etc.)?

There are also a number of apps that can be used to track pain. Some of these can be helpful—find an app that works best for your client. With apps, I find that there can be an addictive quality to logging, whether it is a diet tracker or a pain tracker. Review this with your client, and if you are unable to find one that is a fit, old-school pen and paper works just fine!

Summary

Chronic pain is pain that lasts for three months or more, and it is the leading reason that people seek medical attention. Pain is subjective and everyone experiences it differently, so we need to ask questions. Due to the stress it causes, chronic pain is a risk factor for suicidal ideation. It is important to assess your clients for their eating disorder symptoms, level of pain, and suicidal ideation as part of your normal practice. It can be high risk for someone to have a high pain threshold and tolerance for pain as they ignore important signals for danger. Work with your clients to ensure they have a plan for their pain flare that includes physical and emotional support. The next chapter will build on the ideas of chronic illness and pain and how they relate to body image.

References

Cleveland Clinic. (2024, September 9). Chronic pain. https://my.clevelandclinic.org/health/diseases/4798-chronic-pain
National Institute of Mental Health (NIMH). (2024). Ask Suicide-Screening questions. www.nimh.nih.gov/sites/default/files/documents/research/research-conducted-at-nimh/asq-toolkit-materials/asq-tool/screening_tool_asq_nimh_toolkit_0.pdf

PainScale. (n.d.). The relationship between chronic pain and anxiety. www.painscale.com/article/the-relationship-between-chronic-pain-and-anxiety#:~:text=Anxiety%20can%20increase%20chronic%20pain%20in%20a%20few,lead%20to%20a%20decrease%20in%20movement%20and%20activity

Santos-Longhurst, A. (2018, November 29). Types of pain: How to recognize and talk about them. Healthline. https://www.healthline.com/health/types-of-pain

Themelis, K., Gillett, J. L., Karadag, P., Cheatle, M. D., Giordano, N. A., Balasubramanian, S., Singh, S. P., & Tang, N. K. (2023). Mental defeat and suicidality in chronic pain: A prospective analysis. *Journal of Pain*, *24*(11), 2079–2092. https://doi.org/10.1016/j.jpain.2023.06.017

Torres, B. (2022, June 9). Pain tolerance and pain threshold. Novus Spine & Pain Center. https://novusspinecenter.com/blog/pain/pain-tolerance-pain-threshold

Chapter 4

The Intersection of Body Image and Chronic Illness

When I heard the word *deformity* as a pre-teen, it changed my life, as I discussed in Chapter 1. When we are young, and our personalities and views of ourselves are developing, the words we are told about ourselves become our reality. In Erikson's "early school years/industry vs. inferiority" stage of development, we become aware of ourselves and our separateness from others (Vankerckhoven et al., 2022). The words we hear from others, whether positive reinforcement or negativity, become a part of how we see ourselves.

Childhood is a time when we develop our core beliefs about ourselves. Body image associated with a disability often goes unnoticed, and the impact of chronic medical conditions on eating disorders and body image is something that we have barely scratched the surface of. If there is illness or injury during this phase of development, the disruption of self and body image disturbance is greater. Many develop an eating disorder due to their body image disturbance and being in a body that "doesn't work the way it is supposed to."

Children in this stage learn to compare themselves to others. We see this drive to compare at all ages, everywhere—in our workplace, families, possessions, and especially in social media. However, at this age, the comparisons can change the sense of self and trajectory of life values and decisions. Developing skills as we grow and mature also lays the foundation for self-esteem, self-worth, and potential future accomplishments. If that is disrupted, it will have a ripple effect in all future stages of development.

We will often see the drive to compare along with self-objectification.

What Are the Risks of Self-Objectification?

Self-objectification is examining and judging your body based solely on its appearance. This is a risk factor for body dissatisfaction, disordered eating,

DOI: 10.4324/9781003500254-6

and other body image concerns. Self-objectification is linked to appearance in comparison to others. When we reach adolescence, we are at a much greater risk of comparison to others. During this phase, body image may become more important than any other part of self or personality; it becomes a dominant characteristic of identity. Adolescence is often characterized by an identity crisis, a lack of sense of self, and confusion over roles.

Adolescence serves as a bridge from childhood to adulthood. Trauma, lack of support, and disruption of self lead to confusion and disturbance in one's sense of self and direction leading into adulthood. This is where we will often start to see more disordered thoughts around the body and food. Without a true sense of self, we find it in the things that start to define us, whether that is body size, illness, social relationships, or an eating disorder diagnosis.

If, during this stage, the sense of self and body are disturbed by illness, it can interrupt this process and lead to increased body dissatisfaction and distress. The earlier the onset of illness, the more significant the disruption to the sense of self. This is ideally the time of intervention by mental health professionals. If, when diagnosed with an illness, a patient starts therapy to adjust, grieve, adapt, and receive validation, the disruption to the sense of self could be less severe or less likely to occur.

The words our medical providers and families use during childhood and early adolescence become our internal voice. That can be a positive, supportive voice or an inner critic, likely somewhere on the spectrum in between. Family members and medical and mental health providers can interrupt the inner critic early to shift the trajectory, not only of the sense of self but also the likelihood of comorbid mental health concerns, including an eating disorder, depression, body dysmorphia, and so on. I will offer suggestions later in this chapter on how to use helpful language with clients.

I would like to share more about my personal experience to provide an example of how words shape children and adolescents. By definition, scoliosis is a skeletal deformity. Once I heard the word *deformity* surrounded by other descriptions of my condition, I started associating very negative thoughts toward myself: *ugly, gross, disgusting, unlovable*. Those words became my core beliefs about myself. Internalizing words, such as deformity, during these critical stages, can lead to a perfect storm in the formation of an eating disorder as well as other comorbid psychiatric issues. At a young age, that language greatly increased my body dissatisfaction and forever changed how I would see myself. That word felt like whiplash. It wasn't a gradual change in my view of myself and my body—I got hit by a truck and my world was shattered. Who I was and thought I could be disappeared. I was now *deformed*—that is who I was and who I would always be.

Functional Aesthetic Body Image

Studies linking chronic illness to eating disorders illustrate how the two conditions relate. In a 2019 study, Thomas et al. (2019, pp. 81–92) explored body image as it relates to functionality in women with visible physical disabilities. The study found that women with visible physical disabilities have a higher body image dissatisfaction and a higher risk for eating disorders than the general population.

The field is now exploring *body functionality as a part of positive body image. Functional aesthetic body image* is defined as "how I look to myself and others while engaging in activities and functions." A study interviewed women up to age 55 with congenital or acquired disabilities with a 13-question qualitative questionnaire; questions focused on body image and body functionality, as well as how their disability impacts the way they view their appearance (Thomas et al., 2019). Marie reflected that "body image is how good, or bad, you feel in your own skin." Catherine defined body functionality as "having your body be able to do what it needs to get through the day." Nine women described fluctuations in their body image that aligned with fluctuations in their health symptoms, whether it was functionality or pain.

I can relate to all of this and recently noticed that I have more issues with my body image when I have an increase in pain or a decrease in functionality. To combat my negative feelings about my body functionality, I realized that I tend to change my clothes often so I can put on a happy face and project a body image that best represents how I want to feel or feel most of the time when I am not experiencing a flare or limitation. Looking better doesn't make me feel better; however, I feel that it gives others the illusion that I am okay. At this stage of my journey, I am not changing my clothes because I am self-conscious about my size or level of attractiveness, but I do so to feel comfortable in the outside world (and to myself).

Smile and Look Pretty for the Pictures

September 7, 2024—This week, I changed my clothes a few times because I was in physical pain, not because of appearance. When I say "smile and look pretty for the pictures," I mean I need to look professional instead of just lying in bed. I noticed that when my pain is worse, I might change my clothes a lot one day and then not engage in that behavior at all for months. This isn't typical for me, but it shows how my pain affects how I view my body.

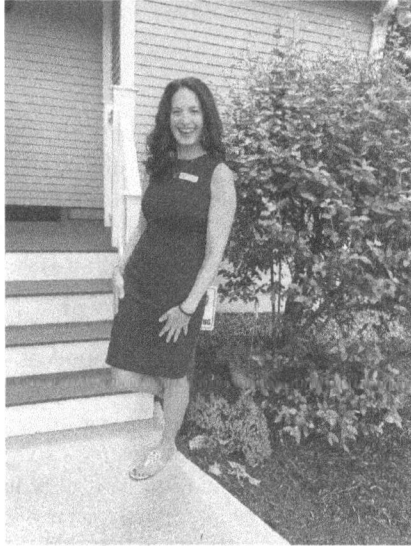

Smile and Look Pretty for the Pictures

Body Image Versus Body Reality

When we assess our clients, *it is important to validate that their body image disturbance is real and not a distortion*. Take it from my 15-year-old self, for example. My body image was distorted as I thought that I was much bigger than I actually was. I did not see that I was slowly disappearing and getting smaller. And my body image was also disturbed. I did, in fact, have a curved spine with a rotation giving me a thoracic kyphosis, also known as the rib hump. To me as a teenager, my body was different from my peers', and it caused me to think poorly about myself. The language my doctors used during my treatments did not help matters.

More than a quarter century later, I was at a scoliosis conference in May 2024 and was able to chat with physical therapists from around the globe. Instead of "deformity" and "rib hump," they used words like *asymmetry* and *uneven*. Using neutral words around clients is very helpful, as it does not stigmatize the "defect" or "deformity" and gives a language to use that is not harmful. When I was 15, my perception of my size was distorted; however, my curve and asymmetry were real. Clothes hung differently on me because of my uneven waist and hips. I tried to wear baggy clothes to try to hide both my size and my curve.

Still Managing How Clothes Fit

October 2, 2017—This was a work dinner that I hosted and was a great event. I loved that dress, and I was really proud of how we set up the restaurant and it was really successful event. And then when I look back at this picture, the only thing I could notice is that my belt and my waist was uneven, and that is something I just was always so self-conscious about. So my uneven waist and hips definitely overshadowed how I felt when I saw this picture.

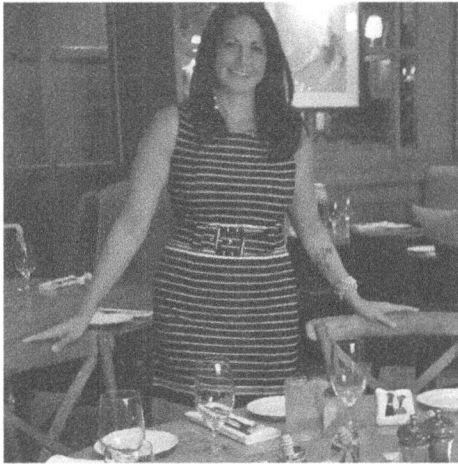

Still Managing How Clothes Fit

The confluence of chronic illness with body image disturbance and distortion can be challenging to untangle as clinicians and even as individuals experiencing the situation. Are we addressing the real disturbed body image due to disease, deformity, or illness? Are we also tackling the body image distortion related to the eating disorder? This is where it is important to talk about body ideal and body reality.

- Our *body reality* is our body as it was created—height, organs, hair color, genetic makeup. It can change as a result of illness, injury, or surgery.
- *Body ideal* is what we learn from culture, friends, and family, and is often where the war with ourselves and our bodies stems from. My family focused on thinness and weight loss, the belief that you must be

thin to be loved. Although we didn't have social media then, that didn't stop me from putting pictures of supermodels on my walls, wishing and hoping that I would look like them. That was my body ideal.

My body reality changed throughout my lifespan and continues to. Everyone's body changes as a result of aging and normal degenerative changes. As I told my story in the first chapter, you saw how my body changed over the years: diagnosis of scoliosis, being braced, surgeries at 26 and 30 years old, then again the complex spine fusion when I was 43. My body reality changed again in 2023 when I broke my wrist and clavicle in an obstacle course race. I have more titanium and a new scar.

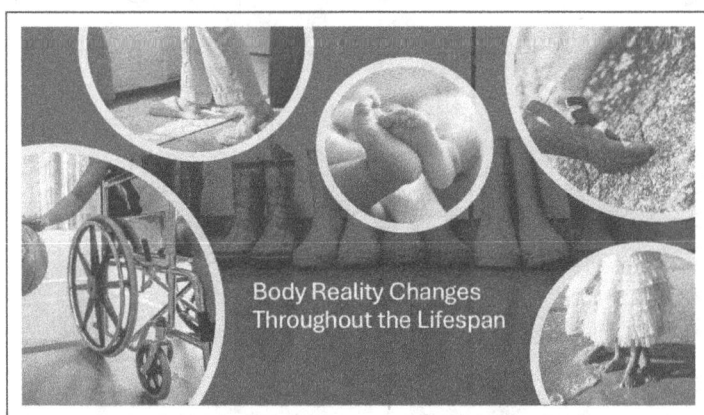

Body Reality Changes Throughout the Lifespan

Unsolicited Commentary on Body Changes

One thing I didn't anticipate was the number of body comments I received from others after my spine fusion surgery. My weight was essentially the same after my fusion; however, my body looked different. My hips and ribs were in a different place, my shape was different, I no longer had my rib hump, and I gained an inch in height. Many people made comments that I looked skinny. I never liked that word and I was surprised that people freely made these comments. This prompted me to do a side-by-side comparison of my back pre- and post-op. I did this to highlight the changes to show that, even though I looked different, I had not lost weight. I was surprised that people thought that it was okay to make comments about my size. I found these comments hurtful; the reason for my surgeries was to restore my quality of life, not to improve my appearance.

My Curvy Body

I've always felt self-conscious about my appearance and longed to look like the girls at the pool with their straight spines. My back is curved, and I am soft around the middle, but I embrace it. Despite the pain and heartache my curvy body has brought me, it has also opened doors to connect with amazing people and challenge myself in ways I never imagined. My journey is a testament that our struggles can lead to a deeper sense of connection.

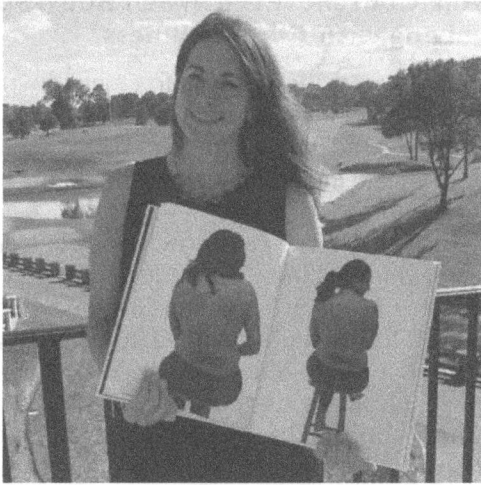

My Curvy Body (Lubar, 2019)

At the SOSORT (International Society on Scoliosis Orthopaedic and Rehabilitation Treatment) conference in May 2024, I wore a dress to show off my spine scar, and it was a wonderful experience. It was empowering. When someone offered to take photos of my back, I took the opportunity, and it turned out better than I could have imagined.

However, we need to be careful when we make comments about people's scars because they can feel invalidating. People often say things like "your scar tells a story," "it shows that you are a survivor," or "scars are tattoos with better stories." While I appreciate these sentiments, scars can be distressing, and using a generic feel-good reply to someone with a scar can completely invalidate their experience.

I went to see Dr. Jordan Wang to help with the scar on my wrist after surgery. It was painful, so I had a laser treatment. We began to discuss scarring and laser treatments to help with the appearance. That led to a conversation about scars from self-harm. He told me that he has had many patients who have seen him to reduce the appearance of these scars. While some people are happy to share about them or get cool tattoos over them, he said that sometimes we don't need a cool story; sometimes they want to move past them, and that's okay. I loved his perspective, compassion, and understanding of how people can sit with these scars in various ways.

How Social Media Content (Even When Body-Positive) Affects Those Living with Chronic Illness

In today's culture, social media is a driving force of how people see themselves and the world. Clinicians must understand its impact on those with chronic illnesses to provide adequate care. Chronic illness may have unique implications on body image including diminished bodily functionality and potential appearance effects.

Isabel Cunha et al. (2024) created a research study to examine body-positive social media and chronic illness. This study was the first of its kind and was first presented at the Academy for Eating Disorders Conference in New York City in March 2024. This study included 201 participants ages 18–41 with one self-identified chronic illness. Participants were randomized to view chronic-illness-inclusive body-positive content or mainstream body-positive content. These participants were recruited and distributed through social media platforms, primarily Instagram accounts with over 1,000 followers. The framework of this study was through the social comparison theory (Cunha et al., 2024). *Social comparison theory* was created in 1954 by Leon Festinger, and it is the idea that people determine their self-worth based on how they measure up to others.

The researchers found that comparison of idealized images of able-bodied individuals may contribute to poor body image in chronically ill populations. Insufficient representation may have body image implications in those living with an "invisible illness." This can discredit the severity of their condition, leading to feelings of not fitting in.

This may also contribute to feelings of not being sick enough. Someone with an eating disorder, at times, relies on changes in body size as a way to "ask for help" because they do not have the words to express their emotional anguish. They need people to "see" that they are not okay. This is a parallel experience to those with a chronic or invisible illness. When people look at someone with an invisible disability, they cannot "see" that there is something wrong. This leads to feelings of having to justify their illness to others.

Although I have an invisible illness, there are parts of it that are visible to me. I felt envious when I saw pictures of people with straight, "normal"-looking spines. We need to be aware of these nuances. Although others may not have noticed my asymmetries, they were very noticeable to me.

Let's examine some ways clinicians and individuals can assess body image in relation to chronic illness.

Ways to Evaluate Body Image in Those with Chronic Illness

There are several established, research-based tools clinicians can use to evaluate body image in those with chronic illness.

Body Image Disturbance Questionnaire (BIDQ) by Thomas F. Cash and Kathleen A. Phillips

This is my preferred measure to use with clients, even though I don't prefer the word *defect*. This survey most accurately depicts body image not intertwined with disordered eating. Here we are looking at body image as it relates to disability, not disordered eating. We know that in those with eating disorders, body image distortion is often present. We also know that in a client with both an eating disorder and chronic illness, the body image disturbance is separate from body image distortion; however, they can intersect. This can make evaluation and treatment more complex and nuanced.

The BIDQ asks questions about body image disturbance and how it relates to psychosocial functioning. Questions focus on how the physical "defect" has impacted a client's life. This focus can relate to a client's social life, employment, avoidance of activities, and so on.

I would suggest reviewing this scale with your clients. Seeing the word "defect" can be upsetting, so I would recommend reading the questions to your client and working through this together in session. You can read the questions and use whatever word you like in its place. For example: "Please tell me how your scoliosis has impacted your social life. How has your pain and fatigue impacted your career?"

Body Image Quality of Life Inventory (BIQLI) by Thomas F. Cash

In this inventory, clinicians can help clients look at how feelings about appearance and body image impact different parts of life, including feelings in relationships, places of employment, confidence, and happiness. I am in favor of adding this survey to our arsenal because it is generalized and not related to a specific body part or to body image distortion related to an eating disorder. I also feel that there is more room for accuracy with a seven-point Likert scale instead of the typical five, starting with a very negative positive effect to a neutral to a very positive effect.

Functionality Appreciation Scale (FAS) by J. M. Alleva, T. L. Tylka, and A. M. Kroon Van Diest

This scale was created to assess an individual's abilities and how they feel that their body functions. These are important dimensions of body image in addition to actual physical appearance. I appreciate the FAS for its simplicity, directness, and neutrality of questions. This is a questionnaire we should be using in addition to the BIDQ (BIDQ-S for scoliosis-specific patients).

This scale is subjective, and the responses can change over time. It allows a patient to look at their body in a neutral way and think about it as it functions, not as it appears in the mirror. It directs an individual to pause and assess *how they feel* about their functionality, which is different from their actual physical functioning. For example, I might have more limitations now with the emergence or progression of a chronic illness, but I have a new appreciation for my body. This appreciation may change over time, and I may be more grateful for my body now than I was in the past when it was perceived as functioning "better." (See Chapter 15 on joyful movement to understand how this evolution can occur.) Resilience may lead to a changed perception of the value of our bodies and our challenges, limitations, success, and growth.

How This Information Can Help Clients

The scales and questionnaires listed above are useful tools to ask questions that a client may not have considered in the past. If they are in treatment for their eating disorder, body image groups and discussions likely focus on distortion and seeing their body as larger or smaller than it is. Treatment may focus on body dysmorphia and not ask questions about how an individual feels about how their body performs when it "isn't working the way it is supposed to."

I believe that knowledge about oneself and gaining insight are two of the greatest tools individuals have in recovery. When an individual has the correct medical diagnosis, they can create a plan of care with their medical team. The same applies to mental health diagnoses. If an individual has the correct diagnosis, a clinician can then come up with the best plan for them. When I was in treatment for the last time, my therapist took out the DSM and showed me the criteria for PTSD. I fit the criteria for chronic complex PTSD, and while this was a shock, it was also a relief to see, in black and white, what was wrong with me.

These scales can give us a new language, framework, and lens with which to view our bodies. They can help us differentiate between body image disturbance related to illness and what is coming from a place of body dysmorphia or distortion.

Summary

The words we hear about ourselves when we are young become our inner critic. There can be a loss of sense of self when diagnosed with an illness at a young age. It is important to offer support and address body image when a medical diagnosis occurs as well as continued changes as a result of illness. Self-objectification and social comparison are a normal part of development; however, this can be a part of the perfect storm in the formation of an eating disorder, especially when someone has a body that is different from others regarding ability or illness. Body image disturbance, related to illness, is distinct from body image distortion as a part of the eating disorder. We must assess and look at both together. The use of neutral language is useful for both challenges. Many questionnaires are helpful in assessing changes in body image and quality of life as it relates to illness. In the next chapter, we will address these issues related to invisible disabilities.

References

Alleva, J. M., Tylka, T. L., & Van Diest, A. M. K. (2017). *The Functionality Appreciation Scale (FAS)*. www.sciencedirect.com/science/article/abs/pii/S1740144517301948

Cash, T. F., & Fleming, E. C. (2002). *Body Image Quality of Life Inventory (BIQLI)*. https://psycnet.apa.org/doiLanding?doi=10.1037%2Ft07580-000

Cash, T. F., Phillips, K. A., Santos, M. T., & Hrabosky, J. I. (2004). *Body Image Disturbance Questionnaire (BIDQ)*. https://psycnet.apa.org/doiLanding?doi=10.1037%2Ft20989-000

Cunha, I., Nett, S., Lamm, E., & Rodgers, R. (2024). State Effects of Body Positive Content on Social Media Users with Chronic Illness [Review of State Effects of Body Positive Content on Social Media Users with Chronic Illness]. www.sciencedirect.com/science/article/pii/S1740144524001189

Lubar, S. (2019). *SPINES: The Art of Scoliosis*. https://www.bracingforscoliosus.org.

Thomas, E. V., Warren-Findlow, J., Webb, J. B., Quinlan, M. M., Laditka, S. B., & Reeve, C. L. (2019). "It's very valuable to me that I appear capable": A qualitative study exploring relationships between body functionality and appearance among women with visible physical disabilities. *Body Image, 30*, 81–89. https://doi.org/10.1016/j.bodyim.2019.05.007

Vankerckhoven, L., Raemen, L., Claes, L., Eggermont, S., Palmeroni, N., & Luyckx, K. (2022). Identity formation, body image, and body-related symptoms: Developmental trajectories and associations throughout adolescence. *Journal of Youth and Adolescence, 52*(3), 651–669. https://doi.org/10.1007/s10964-022-01717-y

Part 3

Challenges

Part 3 focuses on the challenges faced by individuals living with chronic illness and eating disorders. A clinician should have a broad understanding of how someone with a chronic illness encounters their daily life and overcomes the limitations of their condition. I will share the stories and lived experiences of Karlee, JK, Colleen, and Kiah to highlight how individuals can navigate these challenges and how eating disorders combined with chronic illnesses impacted their lives. I will define invisible and dynamic disabilities, and examine how these conditions affect those who experience them.

Additionally, I will explore the relational dynamics involved, including the concept of interdependence and the necessity of seeking help. The stages of grief can be distinct for those with chronic illnesses, and I will outline these stages and discuss how grief manifests in the lives of those living with chronic illnesses.

The chapters in this section will also cover pre- and postoperative mental health care, including assessment and planning strategies. Furthermore, I will address the implications of eating disorders on surgical outcomes. I will explore medical trauma and its impact on an individual's life.

Each chapter will include relevant research findings and conclude with practical suggestions for clinicians. I also include more of my personal story highlighted in social media posts.

- Chapter 5: Invisible Disability
- Chapter 6: Grief
- Chapter 7: Pre- and Postoperative Mental Health Care
- Chapter 8: Chronic Illness, Medical Trauma and PTSD

DOI: 10.4324/9781003500254-7

Chapter 5

Invisible Disability

"The hardest thing about having an invisible disability is that most people never see what you must do to be as 'successful' as you are"—Anonymous. This is one of my favorite quotes because it describes one of the more challenging aspects of living with chronic illness. These conditions are complex, and they often limit an individual in ways you would not predict. For example, I might be able to run an obstacle course race, but it's really difficult for me to mop my floor. I can climb a rope, but sitting in the car for hours is painful. There often doesn't seem to be a rhyme or reason to physical limitations, which makes it hard for others to comprehend unless they share a similar experience. One of the challenges here is feeling the need to justify to others. I often feel as though I need to explain that I am having a pain flare or that I just had an injection so that I am "allowed" to feel the way I'm feeling. Having a dynamic disability lends itself to internalized ableism. I often feel the need to describe how I am feeling to others regarding changes in pain levels and limitations; it can be frustrating to need to advocate for myself in this way.

The Unseen Side of Chronic Illness

Many chronically ill people have no obvious disability or signs of disease. To those who do not know them or to those who meet them in times of relative well-being, they appear as completely healthy. According to UMass, 10 percent of Americans have an invisible disability (Accessibility.com, n.d.). Many struggle to accept their disability and its challenges as a result of *internalized ableism*.

Ableism is discrimination or prejudice against individuals with disabilities (Merriam-Webster Dictionary, 2024). This line of thinking assumes that everyone should act in a nondisabled way, and any challenges are seen in a negative light. Those with disabilities are seen as less than and inferior in some ways.

DOI: 10.4324/9781003500254-8

Internalized ableism is framing this viewpoint toward ourselves. It shows up in many different ways, and many of us are unaware that we are struggling with this. For example, this occurs when I try to constantly prove myself and my worth. This can lead to me overextending myself with travel or taking on too many commitments. I might think that people won't notice my disability if I am accomplishing so many things. There is something satisfying (and also annoying) when people ask me how I do everything I do. It's as if I'm fooling them—they have no idea what I struggle with on a daily basis because I can "do it all." Yet they have no clue as to what it takes to do it all, and some days I accomplish many things with my laptop while I'm in bed!

I also feel lazy if I need to ask for help, need extra rest, or have to admit that I cannot do something. I often feel guilty if I cancel plans or say no to plans because I need to rest or am in pain. I also struggle with using the word *disabled* to define myself; it's a feeling of not looking disabled or not being "disabled enough." It doesn't help to compare suffering. It is important to acknowledge that sometimes you can't show up for anyone else but yourself and that is okay. Some days, you have just enough for yourself: you need to keep it for yourself and not give it away (see Chapter 13 on spoon theory for more on how an individual can manage energy levels realistically).

Dynamic disability is a newer term; I like this one because it more accurately describes many of us. It means that your level of ability and need for help and assistive devices changes from one day to the next. This idea is more out in the world than ever before thanks to Brianne Benness, who created the hashtag #dynamicdisability to spread this idea on social media; she has a chronic illness and is the host of the *No End in Sight* podcast. Dynamic disability contrasts with *static disability*, which is one that does not change from day to day; examples of this include blindness, paralysis, or limb loss (Reese, 2024).

As a clinician, dynamic disability could cause your client to feel like they don't fit in among their peers and in the settings of their day-to-day lives. I have heard many say that they "aren't disabled enough." A dynamic disability means that your client with a chronic illness can look and feel different every day. Some days, they might have endless amounts of energy and be able to do certain things without assistance, while on other days they may need a wheelchair, shower chair, or assistance getting dressed. These experiences vary from person to person. Additionally, when someone has a dynamic disability and needs that change from day to day, it can be more challenging to ask for support.

These challenges of invisible illness and dynamic disabilities may cause an individual to either prove that they "can do it all" or show the outside world that they have physical limitations with specific symbols. For example, I experienced this feeling after my surgery when I needed a handicap placard. I intentionally wore my bone growth stimulator (it looks like a back brace) into the store. I felt like I would be discriminated against because I wasn't limping and had no obvious signs of a disability. Without seeing my x-rays or my scars, I looked okay.

Just like most things in life, we live in the gray, and we are on a spectrum instead of simply disabled or well. Many people live with varying degrees of illness, wellness, and ability. A clinician needs to keep this spectrum in mind when treating someone with a chronic illness.

The Double Whammy of Chronic Illness and an Eating Disorder

"I don't look sick enough."

How often have we heard that from our eating disorder clients? If they have both an eating disorder and disability, it's a double whammy. This presents so many challenges. They might not feel sick enough and have an even harder time asking for help. They may not ask for help at all because they don't feel as though they have an actual illness or their eating disorder isn't severe enough for them to look sick.

A clinician may encounter a challenging mindset to address in some clients living with both a chronic illness and an eating disorder. For example, someone from a group session I facilitated asked, "Why bother recovering from my eating disorder? I will still be sick." I addressed this question with an example from another participant in an earlier group session, who stated that their chronic illness can be "made less difficult by taking care of myself." She was referring to the fact that although her eating disorder did not cause her disability and her disability did not cause her eating disorder, her quality of life was much better when she was taking care of herself. The client was able to see that when she does not use eating disorder symptoms and supports her well-being, she may need her assistive devices less frequently and will be able to tolerate more movement. Obviously, this means different things to each person. Recovery from illness, injury, and surgery is all "made less difficult" when we are doing what is best for our bodies.

Karlee's Story: Eating Disorder, POTS, Lupus, Endometriosis, and Ehlers Danlos

Karlee has lived, treated, and managed an eating disorder and delayed chronic illness diagnoses for more than half her life. She developed eating disorder symptoms in very early adolescence and did not see the connection between them, her mental health, and her physical symptoms from chronic illness until later in life. She lived in a family that shut down mental health struggles as well as the physical symptoms of her chronic illnesses. Since being diagnosed with several conditions, Karlee has been able to recover from her eating disorder, get answers for her chronic illnesses, and help others experience similar challenges.

When Karlee was ten years old, she was in gym class and running laps around the basketball court when she became aware of how she did not like the look or feel of her stomach. Rather than discuss why she felt this way or connect it to growing up, her mom put her on Weight Watchers when she was 11 years old. Her mother thought this was the way to help her.

She continued having body image issues and developed an eating disorder in her early teenage years. She also struggled with physical symptoms of undiagnosed chronic illnesses. She went into eating disorder treatment in 2016, and the treatment provider stated that her physical symptoms were a part of her eating disorder. However, as her eating disorder symptoms got better, her physical symptoms still persisted. She felt that if her body recovered from her eating disorder, maybe her body would work better, but that did not happen.

Karlee was still struggling with an eating disorder and physical ailments after this initial treatment, and she wanted to "figure it out." Some of her other treatment challenges were due to her family not "believing" in mental health and the need for treatment. But Karlee persisted. At 17 years old, she started to see a therapist, but she did not tell her mom about this. Her therapist recommended that she seek a higher level of care for her eating disorder. Treatment provided her with the structure she needed to get herself on track. While she did not have the support of her family, her best friend's family was a great support to her and even helped with paying for treatment as she did not have health insurance.

She had been suffering from medical symptoms for years, but they got much worse after she was in a car accident in 2019. Head injuries can trigger postural orthostatic tachycardia syndrome (POTS), which was her diagnosis after the accident, though she had suspected it for years. Symptoms of this condition include dizziness upon standing, headaches, nausea, and blurred vision. While eating disorders do not cause POTS, the symptoms could be made worse by eating disorder symptoms. She had a prior diagnosis of Ehlers Danlos syndrome (EDS), and her symptoms worsened after her accident. Often, POTS and EDS are diagnosed together. She also dislocated her shoulder and wrist in the accident.

Months later, Karlee continued to feel sick. In early 2020, at the onset of the COVID-19 pandemic, she was diagnosed with lupus. She had experienced lupus-like symptoms for years, but she was never diagnosed. Often, lupus is characterized by a rash on the face, but she assumed since she was often in the sun because she lived in a southern state that she was always sunburned. She began receiving treatment for lupus on top of POTS and EDS.

On top of these chronic illnesses diagnosed years after symptoms began, Karlee finally started to receive medical treatment for endometriosis as an adult. She always had problems with her period, but since she grew up in a religious family, they did not talk about it, and she did not know that her menstrual issues were abnormal. She had no idea that there was a specialist she could see for this, and she now has a trusted medical provider.

Karlee struggles with the invisibility of her conditions. As she says, "I look okay and can do normal things." Because of this invisibility, Karlee feels that she gaslights herself and often doubts her symptoms and body's messages to care for itself. She acknowledges this is a lifelong struggle.

Today, Karlee is a recovered professional. It brings her great joy to help clients who are struggling as she once did. She likes to be an example of recovered, normal eating. She wants her clients to not think about what they are eating. She feels a sense of great freedom with eating and hopes that her clients and others can achieve the same. Now five years into recovery, she is able to see how her physical symptoms of body image are a result of a flare-up with her eating disorder and not a body image distortion.

She does feel frustrated when her body is unable to do something. When she is having a flare, she may be in bed or not able to walk her dog. Karlee wants to live a healthy, active life as much as possible. She enjoys running— it is her joyful movement—and she has embraced it again as an adult (she was not able to run track in high school because of her eating disorder). She took a break from running to get into recovery from her eating disorder and got back into running with the support of her treatment team. Now she chooses her races based on their snacks, scenery, and medals, and delights in weekend runs with her running buddy where they get waffles after their workout.

Interdependence

A concept in theory and in practice that can help clients with a chronic illness and an eating disorder is *interdependence*. This involves a client's mutually beneficial relationship with other people. It essentially is allowing oneself to be vulnerable with another and the other returning that openness. Although clients with chronic illness often require physical help, they are able to offer support to others, such as emotionally. These relationships apply not only to romantic partnerships but also with friends and family. Anyone experiencing a dynamic illness can benefit from interdependent relationships because they allow for grace and changing situations.

As human beings, we share independence, dependence, support, and vulnerability with others. People in an interdependent relationship are not fully dependent on one another; but they tackle life together. Interdependence means that individuals are leaning on each other; they help each other. Rather than someone assuming the role of caretaker, in an interdependent relationship, the power differential shifts and becomes neutral.

I see this in my relationships with my close friends (see my social media posts in this chapter). To have interdependent relationships, it is essential not to keep score and just know that those in the relationship can rely on one another. Relationships are rarely 50/50 as far as effort and interdependence are concerned; they should vary and flow like a wave throughout days, months, and seasons.

Allowing ourselves to be interdependent in our close relationships will enable us to be more independent in all areas of our lives. Remember that this not only applies to help due to disability—it's for all parts of life including eating disorder support. For example, my dear friend Jessica helped me so much when I broke my wrist, and then later I got to take her to a doctor's appointment and to lunch. We also continue to support one another emotionally. Notice how I said that I "got to" help her. It can bring us joy to support one another, so when you feel like you are a burden, remember that although we may not fully believe it, this brings joy.

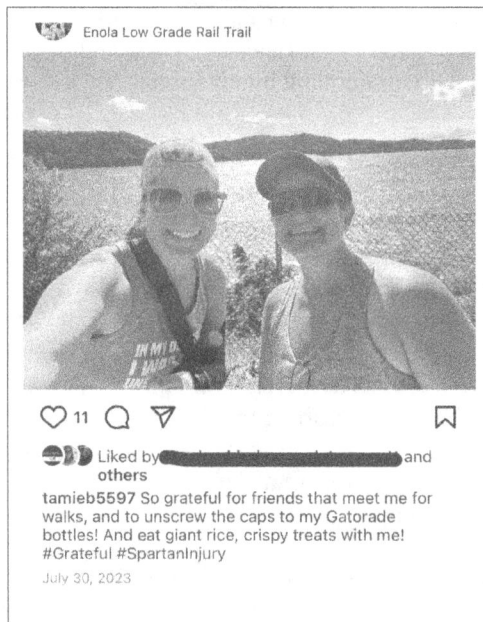

Enola Low Grade Rail Trail

♡ 11 ◯ ▽   ⊓

Liked by [redacted] and others

tamieb5597 So grateful for friends that meet me for walks, and to unscrew the caps to my Gatorade bottles! And eat giant rice, crispy treats with me! #Grateful #SpartanInjury

July 30, 2023

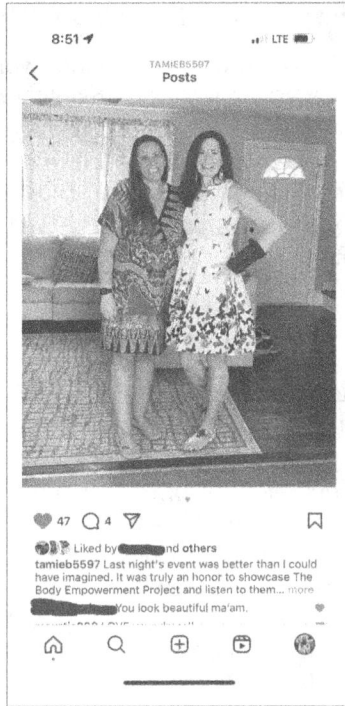

My Interdependent Relationships

Why Are Interdependent Relationships Difficult for Someone with a Chronic Illness?

To feel safe and secure in our world and in our relationships, we need a safe attachment with at least one caregiver in our lives. Research is not available to show the impact of illness on attachment; however, we understand that anything that separates us from that secure attachment can create attachment trauma. Someone who was born with an illness, or diagnosed as a child, has suffered an attachment trauma (Fleming, 2024).

There are many things that cause attachment ruptures including sexual abuse, divorce, or loss of a loved one. We often see attachment trauma associated with those with eating disorders. The impacts of childhood attachment trauma will continue into adulthood. We will talk more about this in later chapters.

If a client has experienced attachment trauma or ruptures, they may find it difficult to enter into interdependent relationships with others. Understanding these challenges can be an important aspect of treatment for a client with a chronic illness and eating disorder.

Building Interdependent Relationships with Others

In theory, interdependent relationships sound wonderful, even idyllic. However, the concept may cause fear and anxiety among your clients, and they might think that they will never trust another again. As clinicians, how can we introduce this concept and work on it in a way that feels safe and manageable? In Chapter 8, we will discuss creating safety and containment. If we have not done this with our clients, we will want to ensure we do this before diving into this topic with them.

Start in Individual Sessions

First, introduce the concept of interdependence and process what it brings up for your client. If you yourself are in recovery, what does this idea bring up for you? During my younger years, I would have responded to this idea with "Absolutely not! There is no way I am going to trust again!" I would then have listed out all of the reasons why trusting someone, especially with me having a disability, is not something I would do again. Do this with yourself before you start working with your clients. Between your own thought exercise and those examples and responses from your clients, the concept of interdependence will become more tangible to discuss with a client. When we know what the fear and struggle are, we can work through those fears and the traumas that caused them. They are valid, so we want to address them and not dismiss them.

Try the Group Dynamic

Clients might not currently have anybody in their lives for an interdependent relationship. Clinicians can work on this in a safe and moderated way in a group setting (see Exercise 5.1 at the end of this chapter for specific prompts to guide a group session). If you have been in a support group, or led one, you see that group is a microcosm for our lives. We see things play out relationally in a group, which is a safe space to work through these issues. For example, if a client is the fixer in their life, they might be the group member that always offers support and advice. If they fear using their voice because they may have been told that they are to be seen and not heard, they might be quiet and not say how they feel.

People have many versions of themselves, and these relational challenges will come up in a group setting. That is one of the reasons that groups are used at higher levels of care and why they can play a vital role in recovery. I love a virtual group to help with this. A participant can remain quiet, then start to use their voice by sharing in chat, and then share out loud! It's a slow progression, and I have seen it help so many gain the trust to use their voice.

As clients gain confidence, they can identify what feels comfortable. Here's an example from a group I led:

> In group on Saturday, you responded to my share about my family visit, and you were able to relate to my share and express similar struggles that come up for you when you see your family. Can you tell me more about what that was like for you? What worked? What didn't work? Are you willing to try this again or in your life outside of a group setting?

Once a client begins to respond in a group session, a clinician can then work to determine how the client can bring interdependence into their relationships, whether that might be with a friend, partner, family member, coworker, or a 12-step sponsor. Clinicians can then teach them how this feels, in a safe way, and work on how to develop that skill in other areas of their lives.

Keep in mind that developing interdependent relationships requires a client to examine their past relationships as well as the relational traumas that they experienced when they were dependent on others. Clinicians begin this work by looking at past relationships and must remember that things will continue to come up for the client throughout this process, so this will remain an essential part of this work. Even though clients are practicing interdependence with safe people (group, sponsor, etc.), triggers will come up, and they need to pause, process, and reflect as they continue to work on these relationships. If a client is struggling with eating disorder symptoms or self-harm urges, clinicians should tread lightly until these symptoms have lessened. However, clinicians should not require someone to be symptom-free before continuing this work. Symptom urges can be vital information to inform treatment goals. Let's continue to be curious about these urges and what symptoms a client may act on.

Be Mindful of Hyper-Independence

A chronically ill client with an eating disorder will likely be *hyper-independent*; I call myself stubbornly independent! Although I am years past my eating disorder, I still struggle with this trait. Originally, it was for self-preservation. However, it can then lead to isolation and more struggle.

Being overly independent may feel safe; however, it is isolating, and biologically and emotionally, we need people to share life with. We also need to acknowledge that *hyper-independence is a trauma response*. Many have been traumatized by their families of origin, by caregivers, by medical providers. Signs of hyper-independence can include the inability to trust, being guarded in relationships, perfectionism, and the inability to ask for help.

Hyper-independence is not a formal diagnosis but can be a part of a PTSD diagnosis. When we have been through a trauma, without needed support, we may compensate by becoming overly independent. This can cause relational issues by not accepting help or even pushing it away. There may then be a confirmation bias: "See, I told you no one listens to me. I knew I was too much." However, that may occur as the result of pushing others away.

Many who are hyper-independent are very distrusting of others, which makes it so difficult to ask for help and even more difficult to receive it. I have personally experienced this in many relationships, and it seems to be most pronounced with family and potential romantic partnerships. The fear of this type of betrayal can cause me to "reject you before you can reject me" or become so hyper-focused on anything that is a potential concern that I become overly critical as a way of self-preservation. Clients discovering this about themselves may find it painful, but it can also be a step in the direction of healing.

How I Struggle and Work Through Interdependence

As I mentioned in my story in Chapter 1, my spine surgeries gave me the courage to leave an abusive relationship. I had a narcissistic, abusive partner for many years, including the times of my greatest struggle and pain leading up to my surgery, as well as during my surgery and recovery. I have experienced similar issues in other relationships as well. I acknowledge that I have a fear of being treated poorly in relationships due to my limitations. When I enter another partnership, this is something that I will have to continue to work through. I have addressed it in EMDR as well as traditional therapy (see more about different therapy options in Chapter 10); however, some things cannot be fully worked through until we are in a relationship.

My race accident shifted my perspective on interdependence and support. My life has changed so much as a result. Living alone, I had no choice but to ask for help. I needed help with everything. So, Ms. Independent could not be hyper-independent. I could only be independent by asking for help. It has also given me permission to continue to ask for help in other ways, such as allowing myself to have a cleaning person every couple of weeks. Cleaning has always been a physical challenge, but I never allowed myself the opportunity to get help with it. With cats, I clean often; however, I no longer have to do the biweekly deep cleaning, and I am so grateful.

Learning how to ask for help can seem daunting, so we need to practice (see Exercise 5.2 for ideas on how a client can practice how to ask for help).

For me, it is easier to ask for help when it is something that I absolutely cannot do on my own, such as needing tangible physical support after surgery. Asking for emotional support can feel more daunting and personal. This is a process and will take time, so be gentle with yourself.

Tools for Fostering Interdependence

Exercise 5.1: Utilizing Community and Group to Explore Interdependence

In *Eating Disorder Group Therapy: A Collaborative Approach*, Carolyn Karoll and Adina Silverman cite many examples of utilizing community and the group experience to practice building relationships and thus interdependence. It is difficult to work on relationships when an individual is not in a relationship, and group can be a safe space to do this. In the development of any relationship, it is important to start slow.

In their group "What's your fear?", clinicians start by asking the group members what fear they have about being in a group. We want to ensure that all group members have the chance to think of their fear. They will then be asked to share their fear aloud. Clinicians should encourage the group to process this together and support one another in identifying and addressing their fears of being in a group.

Here are suggested questions for the group:

1 What was it like to share your fear?
2 What was it like to hear the fears that others shared?
3 Has anyone experienced a similar fear and found strategies to overcome it?
4 Has this discussion and specifically talking about these fears helped you feel more at ease toward them?

Exercise 5.2: Learning How to Ask for Help

Clinicians and individuals themselves can use these prompts to practice how to ask for help from others.

1 Practice in therapy.
   Individuals can start sessions by saying "Today I need ..."
2 Practice in a safe and supportive group setting.
   Individuals can raise their hand and share; it does not have to be lengthy; however, it helps an individual get in the habit of using their voice.
3 Identify a friend to practice with.
   Individuals can talk to their friends to practice; they should inform their friends that this is something they are working on.

Individuals can practice calling/texting a friend to ask for help with smaller things so that they are ready when they need help with something bigger. My close friends and I leave voice notes for each other; this can be a less vulnerable way to ask for help as it is a message and not "live."

Summary

An invisible disability is a disability in which there are no "obvious" signs of illness. Those with a static disability have a disability that will not change or fluctuate; those with a dynamic disability will have shifts in abilities, limitations, and pain levels. Those with chronic illnesses may struggle with hyper-independence where they are not willing or able to ask for help. Working toward interdependence allows someone to become more independent. Interdependence allows individuals to lean on each other in relationships instead of being fully dependent. Individuals can work on interdependence and requests for help in many ways, including individual and group therapy. In the next chapter, we will explore grief associated with diagnosis and life with a chronic illness.

References

Accessibility.com. (n.d.). The truth about invisible disabilities: Statistics, myths, and barriers to Inclusion. www.accessibility.com/blog/the-truth-about-invisible-disabilities-statistics-myths-and-barriers-to-inclusion

Fleming, L. (2024, January 3). The painful effects of attachment trauma. Verywell Mind. www.verywellmind.com/attachment-trauma-7968974

Karoll, C., & Silverman, A. (2024). *Eating Disorder Group Therapy: A Collaborative Approach*. Routledge.

Merriam-Webster Dictionary. (2024). Ableism. www.merriam-webster.com/dictionary/ableism

Reese, B. (2024, July 25). 7 types of protected VA disability ratings explained. VA Claims Insider. https://vaclaimsinsider.com/7-types-of-protected-va-disability-ratings/#what-is-a-va-static-disability

Chapter 6

Grief

Life with a chronic medical condition has many layers of grief that continue throughout the lifespan. Oftentimes, this grief is complicated and hard to understand. I experienced this firsthand following surgical interventions for my scoliosis. After my spine surgeries, I grieved the body that was no longer mine as well as activities, such as riding a bike, that I could no longer participate in.

The Five Stages of Grief

When we think of grief, we might think of the classic five stages of grief: denial, anger, bargaining, depression, and acceptance. Elisabeth Kübler-Ross defined these in her book *On Death on Dying* in 1973 as a means to deal with the experience of dying and acceptance of our own mortality (Kübler-Ross, 1973). Since that time, this framework is something that continues to be used in the processing and treatment of grief in the loss of a loved one as well as many issues in life that cause grief, whether that is divorce, the loss of a job, a health crisis, or another significant loss that is potentially life-altering.

Grief is not a one-size-fits-all experience. The stages of grief are not prescriptive, they do not necessarily occur in this particular order, and not everyone goes through every stage (Mometrix Academy, 2022). However, understanding and discussing the five stages can be beneficial for both clinicians and their clients.

- Denial: In this stage someone might feel overwhelmed and numb and deny the reality of what is happening.
- Anger: Anger is one of the most common emotions of grief. Anger might be directed at a higher power, a medical provider, or anyone or everything. Thoughts of "Why me?" are common in this phase.
- Bargaining: In this phase, people start making promises. "If I get better, I promise to do …" There are many thoughts of "What if?" Someone in this phase may experience feelings of guilt.

DOI: 10.4324/9781003500254-9

- Depression: This is when someone is feeling deeply sad. In the initial months, clinicians aren't typically treating depression because it is situational and often improves within six months.
- Acceptance: This does not mean that grief has ended; however, individuals have started to lean into their new normal. There are likely periods of acceptance followed by cycling back to anger or depression.

Different Types of Grief

Just as an individual will work through the stages of grief uniquely, there are different types of grief a person may experience. As clinicians, it is important to understand the kind of grief your client experiences to meet them where they are for treatment purposes. There are three categories of grief:

- Acute grief: This occurs at the time of loss and is the period when someone is often inconsolable. The onset is sudden, and they will often feel heartbroken and devastated. This phase typically lasts for four to six months.
- Anticipatory grief: This is often characterized by panic, fear of the unknown, and fatigue. This can be anticipation of the loss or potential loss.
- Chronic grief: This grief is unremitting, relentless. This occurs when someone is not able to come to terms with their loss, diagnosis, or prognosis. This is the phase where we may see maladaptive coping skills such as disordered eating, substance use, or suicidal thinking (Mometrix Academy, 2022).

Chronic Grief Is Complex

For those with chronic illness, there are many points in their lives when they can experience grief. Often, this is chronic grief. It can occur at the onset of the illness, with diagnosis, and with each setback or challenge.

Psychologist Jennifer Martin (2015) added two more stages to the stages of grief for those with chronic illness. She looked back on her experience when she was diagnosed with ulcerative colitis and felt that although the five stages are valid, there is a little more to grief with a chronic illness.

Dr. Martin's stages of grief are:

1 Denial: When it comes to illness, denial has a very different meaning than it does for someone who is grieving a loss. Denial of a diagnosis, and its meaning, can be tricky because it can stand in the way of someone getting the medical help they need. Someone may go back and forth with their denial as their diagnosis and/or prognosis changes.

2 Pleading, bargaining, desperation: In this phase, someone may become desperate to do anything that will make the chronic condition go away.
3 Anger: In this situation, individuals may become angry not only with their diagnosis but also with their doctors and their bodies. At times, this anger may look like lashing out at supportive friends or family.
4 Anxiety and/or depression: The grief with chronic illness is grieving the life an individual once had and the future they had hoped for. They may experience anxiety and/or depression about the future and the unknown.
5 Loss of self/confusion: With a life-altering diagnosis, surgery, and changes due to their illness, an individual may not recognize who they are. If they are an athlete, they may no longer be able to compete in their sport. They may not be able to work or travel. They may not be able to care for their family in the way they are accustomed to. They may start to question their value and who they are.
6 Reevaluation of life, roles, and goals: In this phase, individuals are realistically looking at their lives and what they can and cannot do, what they need help with, and what might need to change.
7 Acceptance: This is not when an individual decides that they are OK with their illness, but they are in a place of living in a new normal and navigating what that means for the future.

Similar to the stages of grief for other types of loss, this is cyclical, and someone can vacillate between phases of grief. When there is a new challenge, diagnosis, or struggle, someone may go through all of the phases again. At times, I go right to anger, frustration, and anxiety, and then I am able to reevaluate my life.

Where Grief Can Show Up in Chronic Illness

Grief from Body Changes

Oftentimes, after a surgery or illness, individuals are so grateful for their health that they fail to acknowledge that the changes in their bodies can feel devastating. After my surgery, I often said that my body did not feel like my own. My hips, ribs, and waist were different, I had two feet of scars, I gained an inch in height, and my rib hump was gone. While I was grateful for my surgeries, I could not tolerate the changes in my body. It was upsetting to look in the mirror.

Individuals do not only grieve changes to appearance; even greater grief can come from changes in functionality. It is so important that individuals do not compare themselves to others here. Personally, I had a lot of little limitations that added up. For others, they may have a great loss of mobility and need assistive devices as well as the help of family and friends or in-home nursing care following a procedure or as a chronic illness progresses.

Someone with a chronic illness needs to honor and grieve each change in their lives whether it means no longer being able to ride a bike or no longer being able to work. Each change is significant and important to acknowledge. Later in the chapter, I will talk about some tips for giving space to clients to process these changes, and later in the book I will talk about progressive desensitization to process changes in body (see Chapter 10).

A client with anorexia may grieve the body that they were in and the skinny jeans that they no longer fit into. A client may grieve no longer being able to feel the comfort of a binge. An eating disorder client may grieve the loss of the eating disorder and the purpose it served. An eating disorder and its behaviors may have saved their life in so many ways, and it is normal and often expected to grieve the loss of something that was such a big part of their life. We need to allow space for this.

Grief in Relationships

Relationship dynamics are likely to change as the result of illness. If an individual has a congenital illness, these relational changes can occur if and when there are complications, degenerations, and new limitations. There may be a shift in responsibilities and support needed, whether that is tangible support helping with physical needs or emotional support.

Individuals with chronic illness may struggle to be able to feel fully present in their relationships and may have to make adjustments for their own self-care, which may mean canceling plans or not making plans at all. While friends and family may be understanding of this, individuals may carry guilt and feel the loss of this time with their loved ones.

Additionally, someone with a chronic illness may fear their partner leaving them due to their illness or may fear that they will not be able to find someone to share their life with.

Some relationships do not stand the test of time when there is chronic illness involved. It can often feel like the illness is a third party in a relationship, and it can be difficult to navigate.

Grief of Career

A changing professional identity as the result of a chronic illness is often where someone may feel grief of their sense of self. For many people, their identity is tied to their career. What if they are no longer able to work or are not able to perform the functions of their job? For me, there are many parts of my work that I can do from home, and I have many skills and talents that make up for my sometimes limited ability to travel. But travel is still part of my job. I carry the fear that one day there will be a time when I cannot travel as often and my work may need to change.

For others, their cognition may no longer be clear enough to work, or pain may prevent their ability to work. Grieving a career may not mean that an individual is no longer able to work altogether but that their abilities to perform in the way that they would prefer have changed.

This can be a time when people may say things like "At least you can work from home" or even "It must be nice to work from home." In my experience, people like to tell me the bright side of my situation, and this may shift into toxic positivity. Individuals with chronic illness need the space to grieve and feel the frustration, sadness, and loss of their situation. Then they will need support to help make shifts in their lives. Sometimes they just need to hear "That really sucks, I'm so sorry you are going through this."

Grief and Loss of Abilities

When someone loses the ability to do something in their life because of chronic illness, this can feel like a loss of independence. This may push their edge of wanting to and needing to ask for help. This will look different for everyone. What works for one person may not work for another.

Loss of abilities carries a different meaning, and every loss is significant. Sure, it sounds lovely that I have to get a pedicure because I am no longer able to cut my own toenails. It can be very frustrating to have to explain to them that I have nerve damage and that sometimes I get an ingrown toenail and don't notice until it really hurts. When I do notice, I cannot take care of it myself. This seems like a small thing, but it can be massively frustrating. Another loss is not being able to ride a bike; it doesn't seem like a big deal, but I can no longer do something I really enjoyed. Those little things aren't so little and need space for grief and frustration.

Loss of abilities may include the necessity of assistive devices when someone loses their ability to walk. This can cause tremendous grief, and someone will likely reach a place of acceptance and then cycle back through the stages of grief. There are so many feelings that go along with the need to use a wheelchair or other assistive device. There may be feelings of failure, shame, and guilt for needing more help.

Grief for the Future

Someone with a chronic illness may grieve for the future they may not have due to limitations, a life-altering diagnosis, and acceptance that they may not be able to do everything they had hoped in life. For me, this comes in waves. I try to compartmentalize it as it can be all-consuming to fear what the future may, or may not, hold.

Tips for Clinicians and Clients

When someone is in denial, it is not your role to always "bring them back to reality." Stay in it and be a safe landing space to process this until they can move on to the next phase of grief.

There are times when a reality check is helpful, such as when a client is sure they have gained 10 pounds by adding an apple to their meal plan for that week. If their weight has not changed, this is a great reality check.

You may want to implement dialectical behavior therapy (DBT) skills with clients, including:

- Practicing mindfulness
- Grounding with their five senses
- Urge surfing (see Exercise 6.1)
- Reevaluating life roles and goals (see Exercise 6.2)
- Writing a letter to grieve the loss of the eating disorder

Exercise 6.1: Urge Surfing

This is typically used for a client to ride out the urge to use a maladaptive coping skill such as using eating disorder symptoms or self-harming. The same tactic can work for riding the wave of intense emotions. The intention here is that the intensity of the urge or emotion is time-limited and may last for 15–20 minutes. This does not mean that the feeling subsides at that time; however, the intensity, which can feel unbearable, will lessen at that time. Some people time their urges or intense feelings so they know how long they need to practice grounding skills.

Ask your clients about their grounding and distress tolerance skills. It is important for them to have this on hand and written down or in the notes on their phone as it is difficult to come up with these skills in the midst of an intense emotion or urge. Direct your clients to practice these skills when they are in a grounded place.

Exercise 6.2: Reevaluating Life Roles and Goals

This is something a client will do as they move closer to acceptance. Once they are in acceptance or this new phase of their illness, they can start to examine their role in their family, life, and career, and determine what life will look like now. The hope is that this can be a positive time of exploring new possibilities for career, movement, and family.

For relationships, I recommend that clients bring in their externalized illness. In earlier chapters, I recommended that a client come up with a name for their illness. For example, I can talk about Titanium and its place in my relationships to reevaluate my life and goals.

Profile: JK's Lived Experience

The following is a contribution from JK, who is a yoga therapist, in eating disorder recovery and a long-COVID sufferer. She writes in her own words about grief and what she calls her lifelines.

It was the week of Thanksgiving 2020. I started with a scratchy throat, a low-grade fever, and not feeling well that Tuesday, but felt fine by Friday. I ran and rode my bike that weekend. That Monday, I woke up dizzy and feeling worse, and by the next morning, I was sicker than I had ever been in my entire life. I was in bed for a few months and could not get my energy back. I was not getting better.

I went to a few doctors, a pulmonologist, and infectious disease doctors. I was getting negative COVID tests; however, doctors confirmed that I had COVID. In January 2021, they were just starting to have reports of people not getting better. They started to call it the long haul … they said you should feel better in six months. Now, it's been four years.

My life has been completely transformed and devastated in a lot of ways; my long COVID presents like chronic fatigue syndrome. That doesn't quite capture the depths and despair of this illness. I have been housebound; I don't feel like I fit in the world anymore. I move very slowly; sometimes I will use a wheelchair when I go out. Noise and light around me intensify my symptoms. When I am out for any length of time, I will crash. I can't drive because my cognition isn't clear.

There are so many layers to my grief, and it is constant.

Grief for My Career

I was on a certain path forward, and it has been completely derailed. I am a writer, have a PhD in literature, and am a creator. I own a business; I don't have a single idea in my head. Coming up with new content for my business is incredibly difficult to impossible.

Grief for Being Active and Energetic

I hit my stride in my recovery from my eating disorder; I was able to be active in a safe and fulfilling way, whether going out for a run by myself or with my husband or a hike with my family. I got into rock climbing, and it was a fun challenge. I just wanted to be out in the world. I love a run on a cold morning; I love a run on a hot morning. There isn't a morning that I don't think about going for a run … to be out in the world and get in a little joy that way. This is not possible for me to do right now.

Grief for My Role as a Mother and a Wife

The girls were home from school, and their world was upended because of the pandemic, and I couldn't do anything with them. Years later, it's my greatest grief, just knowing that my situation is affecting them emotionally, and

I can't change it. I am contributing to their trauma, and I can't change it. I can't do all the things I would do with them.

I have grief for my husband. I feel like he deserves better, someone he can go out to dinner with. Being in public spaces really intensifies my symptoms. We only go out on very special occasions, and it is limited. I have to be dropped off at the door and know where all the benches are. It is such a production; there is no freedom. It is just so different from how I know myself to be and how I want to be.

I have found ways to keep things feeling and looking as normal as possible for my kids. Gratefully, my kids have a lot of wonderful friends, and their parents are always happy to take them with them. They are doing a lot of fun things and making great memories. I go to bed with peace in my heart that they are having a full and fun childhood. I go to bed with grief in my heart because I'm not the one doing it with them.

We have found a way to do some things. There is a local small zoo that we have been going to since the kids were tiny. I have to say that I can do this. It will be in a wheelchair, but I can still do it and be a part of it. I am working on trying to see the value and gift in that and acknowledge all of the ways I am present.

I make it my business to keep this house running. I always make sure they know I am making their lunch and dinner. I will always do those things because I need them to feel secure and safe and that I will always take care of them.

Grief for My Future

There is grief for my future and grief about the unknown—what will be and what will not be possible. We're now approaching people's five-year long-COVID anniversary, and there is global grief because millions have been affected and will be affected because this virus still exists. I wish there was more awareness of that. If you get it, the illness could change your life.

Grief for Feeling Like an Imposter

There is grief for feeling like a fraud. I show up for my work and turn it on and turn on the smile. I was not used to relating to my passions that way. It just feels out of alignment with how I have learned to live my eating disorder recovery. I don't want to pretend to be OK if I am not. You learn the people you can be real with, and you learn the people you have to say what they want to hear without betraying yourself.

Finding Purpose

Purpose is such an essential part of eating disorder recovery. It doesn't have to be purpose with a capital P—just something that calls you to do something that keeps you caring. I live by that. I am a certified yoga therapist specializing in working with clients with eating disorders. I work with clients 1:1 on Zoom. We sit in our chairs and do small yoga-inspired practices that can offer tools to support their work in recovery. My work is very purpose-giving.

Lifelines

I have a wonderful therapist who specializes in chronic illness and grief. I have structure to my day, including strolling around my backyard. Being outside is the best way to ground and get quiet—I'm blessed to live in a really beautiful neighborhood. I'm outside even when it's cold. I journal, I do my own yoga therapy, I have heating things all around the house, and I find those comforting. Grounding stones—those tactile, soothing, comforting things. *All of those little things add up. I call them lifelines.*

You have to make space for the grief. I meet it with as much comfort as I can.

Summary

Grief can be very complicated and is chronic in someone with a lifelong illness. The phases of grief are guidelines as individuals continue to move through them. Grief here is layered, and individuals need space to process all of it, including grief of career, future, abilities, and relationships. It is important to have support with this, as denial keeps clients from seeking necessary medical attention. Individuals will likely need to explore their new roles and identity with the support of their therapist and loved ones. JK's story is impactful as she names her grief and her lifelines—how she is able to live her life and get through each day. Staying in the moment and in the day is important to avoid getting caught up in fear of the future. In our next chapter, we will focus on mental health as it relates to surgery, another frequent companion for those with chronic illness.

References

Kübler-Ross, E. (1973). *On Death and Dying*. Routledge. https://doi.org/10.4324/9780203010495
Mometrix Academy. (2022). Five stages of grief [Video]. YouTube. www.youtube.com/watch?v=IH6_AqrgL5E
Martin, J. (2015, April 27). Psychological stages of chronic illness/chronic pain [Blog post]. www.jennifermartinpsych.com/yourcolorlooksgoodblog/2015/4/27/psychological-stages-of-chronic-illnesschronic-pain

Chapter 7

Pre- and Postoperative Mental Health Care

Why Individuals, Clinicians, and Medical Providers Need to Plan Ahead for Pre- and Postoperative Mental Health Care

I want to begin this chapter by stating that surgical procedures are not a universal necessity or outcome for everyone with a chronic illness, so this chapter may not be relevant to all. However, as clinicians, we must be aware that many of our clients with chronic illnesses may face frequent or occasional surgeries and that this can be a large obstacle to their well-being, both physically and emotionally. As you know from my story in Chapter 1, surgeries have been a huge part of my life. My personal experience led me to search for anything that might help medical providers identify mental health issues in patients. I was able to identify one survey that surgeons could use prior to significant medical procedures to determine mental health outcomes. With this information, we can plan ahead for postoperative mental health care.

Prior to my surgery, my anxiety and depression increased, and my doctors and I addressed this with medication. Postoperatively, I was surprised when I started to have PTSD symptoms of hypervigilance, insomnia, anxiety, and mood swings. Although I had many years of therapy under my belt, I did not have a therapist at the time of surgery, before or after. I found it challenging to find a clinician with experience working with someone with a chronic medical condition.

Presurgical Psychological Survey

One goal of my work is to advance the use of mental health support for those with chronic illness, with or without current or past eating disorder symptoms. There is a lack of understanding of this need in the medical community, and this must be remedied to help those living with chronic illness. Let me use an example near and dear to my heart regarding spine

DOI: 10.4324/9781003500254-10

surgery. According to a study by Young et al. (2012) that surveyed 340 spine surgeons, only 37 percent of them used the widely available Presurgical Psychological Screening with their patients. The researchers reported a strong belief regarding the impact of psychological factors on pain relief, adherence to therapy, and return to work. While premorbid mental health diagnosis is not necessarily a determinant of postoperative mental health concerns, those with premorbid psychiatric diagnoses are more likely to develop postsurgical mental health issues (Young et al., 2012).

Here are the reasons mental health should be a consideration in treatment for those with chronic illness. Before surgery, many have suffered years of chronic pain, which is likely to increase their risk of mental health struggles. Prior screening could help physicians and their patients prepare for the possibility of postoperative PTSD, depression, and/or anxiety.

Anyone who has sustained a serious injury or had surgery of any kind (whether or not they have a chronic medical condition) knows the stress that is associated with it. This includes pain, limitations, and needing to ask for help and support. Even if this is a short duration, it causes stress, anxiety, fear of the unknown, frustration, and so on.

We cannot always determine who will struggle after a major surgery, injury, or setback. This is not determined by the type of injury or surgery. Having a mental health diagnosis prior to surgery does not mean that an individual will develop PTSD or depression. If a patient does have a current and significant mental health diagnosis, that could suggest postoperative mental health concerns. A physician, whether or not they use this specific screening, should be mindful in assessing their patients.

Now imagine that the individual has depression, anxiety, and an eating disorder and is heading into surgery. They are going into surgery from a place of deficit, "in the red" so to speak. They are in the red physically, mentally, and emotionally, and they are about to experience something that will require all they have to get through it and recover from it. Going through this from a place of scarcity instead of abundance can lead to a difficult recovery, and other things may arise out of this, such as mental health concerns. I will discuss the nutritional and energy deficits and concerns for those in a later chapter.

Personally, prior to my surgery, I went to physical therapy to get stronger, so I had the physical strength to endure and recover from my surgeries. Why don't we utilize mental health therapy in addition to this? Our minds and emotions also need the strength to endure and recover.

Risk Mitigation for Presurgical Psychological Testing

The good news is that physicians and mental health clinicians do not need to create their own evaluation process for preoperative mental health assessment. There is a new framework for risk identification and mitigation (RIM) with a five-step process from Marek and Block (2023):

1   Identification of risk factors through psychological testing
2   Clinical interviews and review of patient medical records
3   Identification of risk mitigating factors
4   Reviewing data and determination of overall risk
5   Treatment recommendations

This model offers specific recommendations for different surgeries, including organ transplants and spine surgery.

The identification of mitigating factors is critical. There are many unknowns when it comes to surgery, and although someone might have risk factors, there is no definitive way to determine who might have psychological changes and challenges postoperatively. We must determine what can temper risk and improve outcomes. Mitigating factors can serve to soften the impact of surgery or another type of trauma. We know that everyone needs support in place, and these mitigating factors can improve the chances of a positive surgical outcome.

As I described in my experiences in Chapter 5, having tangible and emotional support in place can lead to greater surgical outcomes, treatment compliance, and positive long-term psychological impact.

Surgical Complications from Pre-existing Depression and Anxiety

It is very important that medical providers screen for depression and anxiety prior to a patient having surgery. Some studies show that depression coupled with anesthesia may lead to increased complications including mortality (Ghoneim & O'Hara, 2016). Depression can cause a suppression of the immune system, increasing the potential for postoperative infections or cognitive impairment.

Another study finds that preoperative anxiety can cause increased postoperative pain, increasing the need for pain management/medication. In more severe cases, it may even increase postoperative mortality (Stamenkovic et al., 2019).

These findings may seem extreme; however, they highlight the importance of properly assessing mental health prior to surgery.

Eating Disorders and Surgical Outcomes

There is a lack of research regarding surgical outcomes in those with eating disorders. The research I was able to locate is specific to bariatric surgery; there are many studies on that topic. Eating disorders that are not identified prior to surgery will continue after surgery. Presurgical psychological test-ing is important prior to bariatric surgery for many reasons, including the determination of a current eating disorder. If an eating disorder is identified during evaluation, a plan should be enacted to ensure that the eating disor-der is treated and determine if bariatric surgery is an appropriate interven-tion. Postoperative disordered eating leads to a higher risk of complications and a lower quality of life (Phifer, 2022).

Lack of Training for Mental Health and Medical Providers

Those of us who choose to work with individuals with eating disorders do a lot of postgraduate training, as there is little education for mental health professionals in programs like social work or clinical psychology. Many of us got our start working in treatment programs, which are excellent train-ing grounds. We have many continuing education opportunities available through educational organizations and treatment providers.

Medical doctors have very little training on mental health, eating dis-orders, and what to do when a patient presents to their office with any mental health concerns. In my research, it is no surprise that scoliosis and spine fusion patients are not referred to therapy. I have the privilege of speaking to first-year medical students about eating disorders at one of the Philadelphia-area medical schools for one hour each year. Just one hour! I do my best to highlight the most pressing issues in this clinical area, but I know even my best effort falls short—there is just not enough time. Train-ing in eating disorders is an optional rotation for medical students. Medical providers can find continuing education on mental health concerns, but most training offered focuses on medical interventions.

Suggestions for Medical Providers

At times, surgery is an emergent need, and planning ahead is not an option. Other times, as with spine, hip, and knee surgeries, there is time to plan ahead. My doctor and I did not explicitly discuss the mental health impact of my spinal fusion; however, we did talk about it being life-altering.

I suggest that all specialists screen for depression and anxiety before sur-gery. If someone scores high on the evaluation, there should be a discus-sion and referral to a therapist and psychiatrist.

Screening Tools Medical Providers Can Use Preoperatively

- Beck's Depression Inventory
- Beck's Anxiety Inventory
- Patient Health Questionairre-9 (PHQ-9)

For every major medical procedure, I would start with an assessment—many primary care physicians have patients complete Beck's Depression Inventory to assess for symptoms of depression, as well as Beck's Anxiety Inventory to assess for anxiety. I would recommend that specialists also utilize this screening for all patients who have chronic pain and are planning surgery, and it should be completed post-surgically as well. Assessing a patient's mental health when you are not a mental health provider can be a stressful conversation, even for a surgeon. If a patient completes the survey, at least the doctor has gathered information to express concern. Additionally, PHQ-9 inventory is a nine-question survey used by medical professionals to assess for depression.

Some mental health providers use the Millon Behavioral Medicine Diagnostic (MBMD) to assess factors that may help or hinder a patient's recovery (Clay, 2020). It is an extensive 165-question survey of true/false questions. The breadth and depth of this survey could be daunting and frustrating to a patient who is already feeling overwhelmed, so the shorter inventories may be better.

Suggestions for Clinicians

As a clinician for someone with a chronic illness and an eating disorder, you can help prepare your client for surgery as well. I recommend taking the following actions:

1 Assess your client's mental health prior to surgery utilizing Beck's Depression and Anxiety inventory or the PHQ-9.
2 Collaborate with medical providers to include physical therapists and specialists in your client's treatment and recovery.
3 Implement support strategies with your client.

Exercise 7.1: Help Your Client Move From a Place of Abundance Instead of Scarcity

As a clinician, you can work with your client to move into a more abundant mindset before surgery. Ask questions and help them make a plan for after the procedure, including:

- Identify support people to assist them with emotional needs as well as tangible practical needs, such as help with tasks.
- Bring those support people into therapy to discuss the potential emotional impact of surgery and limitations.
- Identify their needs and how people can help them. This can be tangible or emotional such as:
  - Create a meal train.
  - Create a list of presurgical tasks that they may need help with, such as things to pack, buy, and bring to the hospital.
  - Find people who can assist with household chores.

- Identify coping skills together and agree upon them—help them create a printed list for their people to refer to that is as specific as possible. (Personally, I even created a list of music and movies that I liked so I could listen to or watch them when I was feeling down.)

Activities for Clinicians

There are a lot of strategies clinicians can use to help their clients prior to surgery. Here are some ideas:

- Identify presurgical goals that include getting stronger physically and emotionally, heading into battle. Use SMART goals to help your client identify achievable goals pre- and post-op. These goals are specific, measurable, achievable, realistic and timely.
- Use mindfulness practices. There are specific practices that can be used in times of anxiety and pain.

  - In a study on mindfulness-based interventions (MBIs) in total joint replacement patients, MBIs didn't just decrease pre- and postoperative pain, pain intensity, and unpleasantness. Mindfulness coupled with decreased pain also led to decreased pre- and postoperative anxiety and improved postoperative physical healing and performance (Hanley & Garland, 2022). This study also included cognitive behavioral pain psychoeducation as well as mindfulness of breath and pain.

- Implement cognitive behavioral therapy (we will review in greater detail in later chapters).
- Determine your client's mitigating factors:

  - Who are your support people?
  - What people do you need to set boundaries with, keeping only positive relationships at the forefront?
  - What are your personal strengths and coping skills?
  - What skills can you utilize when recovering from surgery?

When I returned for my follow-up appointment, roughly 4–5 months after my spinal fusion, I was noticeably depressed. My doctor asked if I was okay, and I said that I was struggling but that I was "fine." Thankfully, my doctor knew better and probed me a bit more about my mental state.

What do I mean by "noticeably depressed"? For me, it meant that there was no light in my eyes, no smile (not even a forced one), fatigue, pale skin, and lack of eye contact. (Keep in mind that someone may never "look depressed.") For me, it also included symptoms like isolation, lack of sleep, disinterest in spending time with friends, a feeling of dread, the feeling that things were never going to get better, and trouble concentrating.

I have struggled with depression for most of my life. A life of chronic pain and an abusive relationship, in addition to other life stressors, were the perfect storm for me to continue to have an increased struggle after my spine fusion. You can refer back to Chapter 1 to learn more about my personal journey.

My Personal Experience with Postoperative Depression

By July 2023, I was feeling a lot better leading up to my race accident. I had gotten out of an abusive relationship and was surrounded by supportive friends and family. After the surgery, the recovery process was pretty tough, with mental ups and downs, mood swings, and more anxiety than usual. Thankfully, my depression didn't get worse. I've also been in therapy since leaving that relationship, including EMDR, which really helped me deal with all this stress.

In searching for a picture to accompany this post, I realized that true depression often remains unseen, hidden from the naked eye. Yet, despite the many pictures of me smiling, I know that strength and resilience shine through even the toughest struggles.

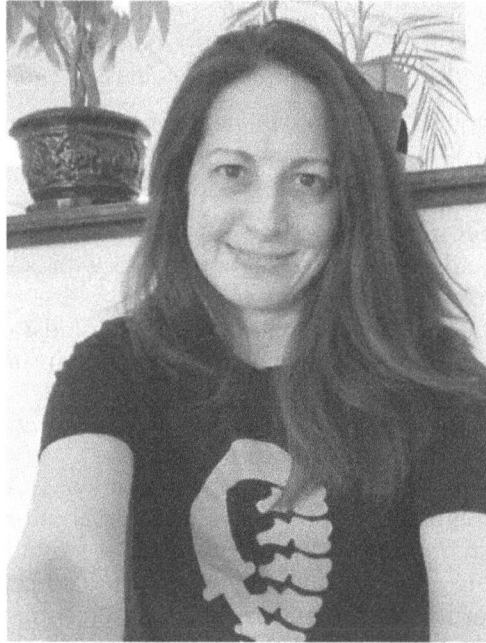

My Personal Experience With Postoperative Depression

Summary

Presurgical psychological testing can help us identify the potential for mental health challenges following surgery. Understanding these risks can help us better prepare for surgery and postoperative outcomes. Pre-existing depression and anxiety can lead to postoperative complications and increased pain. The recommendation is that medical providers screen for anxiety and depression and collaborate with the patient's therapist. Clinicians can help clients prepare by utilizing SMART goals, CBT, and mindfulness, and assessing for mitigating factors. In the next chapter, we will discuss PTSD.

References

Clay, R. A. (2020). *How psychologists prepare patients for surgery.* https://www.apa.org/monitor/2020/09/ce-corner-surgery

Ghoneim, M. M., & O'Hara, M. W. (2016). Depression and postoperative complications: An overview. *BMC Surgery, 16*(1). https://doi.org/10.1186/s12893-016-0120-y

Hanley, A., & Garland, E. L. (2022). Single-session, preoperative mindfulness-based interventions for total joint arthroplasty patients: Pre- and postoperative outcomes from three randomized clinical trials. *Journal of Pain, 23*(5), 34. https://doi.org/10.1016/j.jpain.2022.03.132

Marek, R. J., & Block, A. (2023). *Psychological Assessment of Surgical Candidates: Evidence-based Procedures and Practices.* American Psychological Association. https://doi.org/10.1037/0000346-000

Phifer, A. (2022, February 23). Eating disorders and bariatric surgery: How they intersect [Blog post]. Baylor College of Medicine. https://blogs.bcm.edu/2022/02/23/eating-disorders-and-bariatric-surgery-how-they-intersect

Stamenkovic, D. M., Rancic, N. K., Latas, M. B., Neskovic, V., Rondovic, G. M., Wu, J. D., & Cattano, D. (2018). Preoperative anxiety and implications on postoperative recovery: What can we do to change our history. *Minerva Anestesiologica, 84*(11). https://doi.org/10.23736/s0375-9393.18.12520-x

Young, A. K., Young, B. K., Riley, L. H., & Skolasky, R. L. (2012). Assessment of presurgical psychological screening in patients undergoing spine surgery. *Journal of Spinal Disorders & Techniques, 27*(2), 76–79. https://doi.org/10.1097/bsd.0b013e31827d7a92

Chapter 8

Chronic Illness, Medical Trauma, and PTSD

In Chapter 7, I explored the mental health impacts of surgery related to chronic illness. This chapter will continue to consider mental health in those impacted by chronic illness by exploring mental health challenges following medical procedures. I discuss medical trauma, posttraumatic stress disorder, and medical traumatic stress and how it can impact individuals by sharing my own personal experience as well as the experience of a colleague. Clinicians need to be aware of these deep-seated traumas to help treat their clients experiencing chronic illness. Often, body image issues and eating disorders can result from these traumas, even those that happen in early life.

What Is Medical Trauma?

Medical trauma is the mental, emotional, psychological, and physiological impact of trauma, or a negative experience, in a medical setting, whether that is trauma at the hands of a medical provider or from a life-altering diagnosis, an accident, an injury, or significant surgery. An individual can also experience medical trauma if they have a chronic medical condition and have spent years in a medical setting. The experience may involve illness, pain, invasive or frightening procedures, and distressing or dismissive medical treatment.

Other health-related factors and medical events that can cause medical trauma include:

- Being on dialysis
- Having chronic pain
- Undergoing surgery
- Experiencing medical complications as a child
- Experiencing cancer
- Being intubated
- Having a Cesarean birth

DOI: 10.4324/9781003500254-11

What Is Posttraumatic Stress Disorder?

Experiencing medical traumas can lead to *posttraumatic stress disorder* (PTSD). For example, one in eight heart attack survivors will develop PTSD following their cardiac event, and 20 percent of spine fusion patients suffer from postsurgical PTSD (Oregon Health & Science University, 2012). It is more commonly known for PTSD to occur after a single life-threatening event (such as a shooting or car accident), but cancer is often associated with medical trauma and PTSD (APA, 2020).

Symptoms of PTSD related to medical trauma include:

- Hypervigilance
- Anxiety
- Depression
- Nightmares
- Sleep disturbance
- Flashbacks
- Fear of the future
- Intrusive thoughts
- Fear of entering medical settings

As defined by the American Psychological Association (2020), PTSD symptoms fall into four categories:

Intrusive thoughts: An individual may experience repeated intrusive thoughts and memories or flashbacks of the actual event; their memories may be so vivid that it feels as if they are reliving the event.
Avoiding reminders: Individuals may avoid people, places, or anything that reminds them of the actual event, including talking about the event and how they feel about it.
Negative thoughts and feelings: Individuals may experience ongoing fear, distorted beliefs about oneself, guilt, shame, less interest in previously enjoyed activities, and less interest in connecting with others.
Arousal and reactive symptoms: Individuals may experience irritability, angry outbursts, heightened startle response, difficulty concentrating, disturbed sleep or behaving in a self-destructive manner.

My personal experience led me to want to learn more, so I created a survey to explore the experiences of others. My survey *Mental Health and Body Image Survey in Adults with Scoliosis and Spine Fusion* was shared on social media in 2019. The aim of this study is to examine scoliosis and spinal fusion patients and the associated mental health concerns and psychiatric comorbidities. The additional aim is to discover if patients had the mental health support needed to manage their diagnosis and treatment, what type of support they received, and if a medical professional recommended psychological support. Methods include an anonymous web survey of 185 adults with a scoliosis diagnosis, 80 percent of which have had a spine fusion surgery. Thirty-seven percent of patients were diagnosed under the age of 12, 50 percent were diagnosed between 12 and 18 years of age, and the remaining respondents were diagnosed over 18 years of age. The survey included questions regarding mental health conditions and body image distress as well as postoperative psychological changes.

Results:

- 57 percent experienced symptoms of depression after scoliosis diagnosis.
- 80 percent of adults surveyed stated that they did not feel that they had adequate postoperative mental and emotional support.
- 20 percent of spinal fusion patients reported symptoms of depression.
- 16 percent of patients reported symptoms of PTSD.
- 30 percent of patients reported symptoms of anxiety.
- 66 percent of patients experienced feelings of being different and feeling self-conscious about their appearance after their scoliosis diagnosis and after spinal fusion surgery.
- 99 percent of patients reported that their medical team did not refer them to a mental health professional.

Lived Experiences of Medical Trauma, PTSD, and MTS

To put these issues into a context of chronic illness and disordered eating, I share my story, as well as the story of my friend Colleen. These personal experiences may help clinicians understand the layers of trauma encountered by individuals and provide insight into how to best treat clients experiencing medical trauma, PTSD, and MTS related to their chronic illness and disordered eating.

I Was Injured by a Medical Provider

I was injured by a medical provider who had access to all of my medical records. My physical therapist, at the time, had been working with me on neck pain that was not improving, so she felt that chiropractic could help decrease my pain. Upon meeting with this chiropractor, we agreed that she would only touch my neck and not adjust any part of my spine that is fused. My spine is fused from T10 to S1 and is effectively a fixed structure.

She adjusted over the fused area, and I told her that I was concerned; it scared me. She said that it was fine because she did not use much force. I returned for the second visit that week, and by the following night, I was in the emergency room with severe pain. I was sent home with some pain medication, and the next day, the pain was to a level that I had not experienced since my spine surgeries. I went back to the emergency room and was assessed for every possible concern. I called my spine surgeon and was able to see him that week. I was diagnosed with a costovertebral joint injury in my thoracic spine.

The costovertebral joint is where the rib and vertebra connect. When the chiropractor adjusted me over my fused spine, something had to move, as my spine could not. It caused pain that was terrifying and led to a very long recovery, as documented below. This injury impacted my work, my relationship, my self-care, and my sense of self, and left me questioning my reality.

When I reached out to the chiropractor to express what had happened, she was dismissive of my experience by saying that she did not adjust too hard and that it must be because of my physical activities.

Compounding the medical trauma was being left in the emergency room by my partner. When we are afraid and in pain, we need our people with us, even if it is to watch terrible shows on the small emergency room TV or to simply hold our hand. This event ultimately led me to choose to leave that relationship. Needless to say, this event greatly affected my physical, emotional, and spiritual well-being.

Update Following Medical Trauma

Thank you all for your kind words and well wishes yesterday! Here's a quick update: I tried many methods to relieve my pain, including heat, ice, a TENS unit, ibuprofen, stretching, and even a muscle relaxer, which I usually don't use. Sadly, my condition worsened. I struggled to walk a few steps without crawling and feeling very nauseous, so I went back to the ER. They initially looked for all possible causes and ran several tests. The good news is that I'm healthy, but we still don't have clear answers. I think seeing a chiropractor might have caused some of my problems. Chiropractic care is a debated topic in the scoliosis community, but I wanted to try it to improve movement in my neck. I really appreciate the doctor and the caring nurses and staff at UPMC West Shore for their help. After taking some pain medication and steroids, I was able to walk a bit, so I went home late last night. Now, I will rest, take my medication, and go to physical therapy tomorrow.

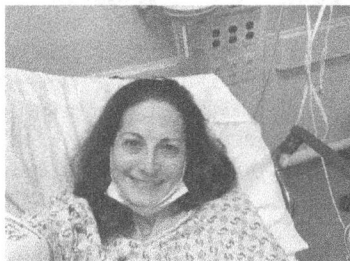

Update Following Medical Trauma

Doing What I Can While Dealing With Medical Trauma

September 11, 2022—Today I walked a 10 K! (Then 1 mile walk back to the car). 5 weeks ago I was in the ER unable to walk. I have a long road ahead of me but walking is one thing I can do that doesn't cause extra pain! So grateful to my friend for walking and talking with me! So much fun!!

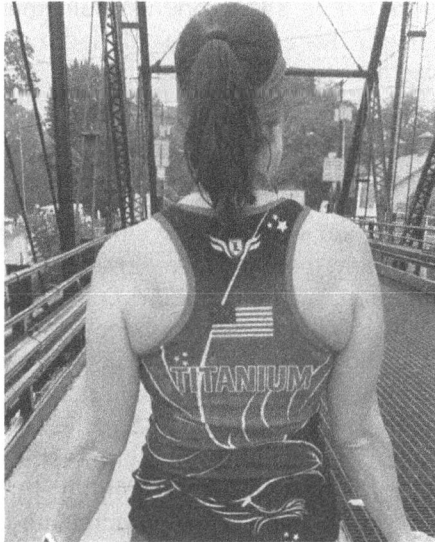

Doing What I Can While Dealing With Medical Trauma

Profile: Colleen's Story—Gratitude in Motion

I met Colleen at a book signing with the women's triathlon club, West Chester Women's Multisport LLC, in the early days post-op from my spine fusion, and I was feeling hopeless about competing ever again. Her strength through adversity, gratitude, grit, and love come through in everything she does. That was a glimmer of hope for me, and I will forever be grateful for her. I share her experience of living with chronic illness, experiencing medical trauma, and finding acceptance from her book *Gratitude in Motion* (2018).

> Lupus isn't easy to diagnose, and usually gets named only by the process of eliminating all the other likely options. On top of that, I was also diagnosed with cryoglobulimenia, a rare condition where abnormal

proteins clump together in my blood vessels in cold weather and cause the plasma to thicken like syrup. All I can tell you is that with all these things combined, this was a dark period in my life. I now knew I had multiple serious and incurable health conditions, including an autoimmune disease, and that any of them could actually kill me. It was work to get myself out of bed and moving each day, to remind myself that it would do no good to stay stuck in despair. I had to find something positive to motivate me.

(Alexander, 2018, pp. 66–67)

In addition to these conditions, Colleen also had a prior history of brain surgery due to Chiari malformation.

On top of these medical conditions, on October 8, 2011, Colleen was riding her bike home from work and was run over by a freight truck. She flatlined twice and required over 70 blood transfusions and numerous surgeries. This caused medical trauma and PTSD, even with a supportive partner by her side.

Sean didn't want to leave my room at all. He watched everything that was happening with me and tried to be my best advocate. The first time he saw me trying to scream was awful for him. During a wound change, my eyes were screwed shut and my mouth was open in a screaming position, but no sound came out. It happened several times a day.

(Alexander, 2018, p. 92)

Her symptoms continued even after the initial stage of her recovery.

The nightmares didn't end once I became aware of what was happening to me; if anything, they intensified. I was on the edge all the time and couldn't win: When I was awake, I could feel all the pain of the injuries and the wound changes. When I was asleep, my mind flew off into horrific imagery.

(Alexander, 2018, p. 98)

Despite the positivity of others, Colleen continued to despair about what had happened to her.

But one thing several people said started to grate on me: "At least you're alive." "At least I'm alive?" I feel like I'm having one long panic attack, my body is torn apart, my husband is sleeping in a recliner instead of next to me in our bed, dozens of strangers have touched my naked body, I'm having unrelenting nightmares … there was not "at least" anything. Every sentence that began with "at least" felt belittling. I couldn't listen to the bright side of anything—it all felt phony. I was just trying to make it through each day, and I did not feel grateful for anything.

(Alexander, 2018, p. 114)

Colleen had trouble looking at her body following the bike accident and her many, many medical procedures, but she experienced an unexpected, powerful moment of gratitude one day. One of Colleen's numerous surgeries was to repair Clyde, her kidney (of *Bonnie and Clyde*—Bonnie was the good kidney, and Clyde was the bad one).

> The next day I stood before the mirror giving myself a sponge bath. Tears welled in my throat at the sight of my naked body, already so disfigured, now bandaged up in four new places where there would be four new incision scars. I stared at my cane handle and my bandages and I remembered to be thankful again, for the surgical team, the nurses, Sean, my friends and family, and for my own imperfect yet still functional body.
>
> (Alexander, 2018, p. 235)

With the love and support of others and through her own painstaking, introspective journey, Colleen found peace despite her difficult circumstances.

> That's where I tried to focus: the love. It was all around me, from the strangers who had saved my life to the lifelong friends who were checking in with my family every day. It's what kept me going even after I thought I couldn't fight anymore. I was in for a long and agonizing journey, but I was never in it alone.
>
> (Alexander, 2018, p. 102)

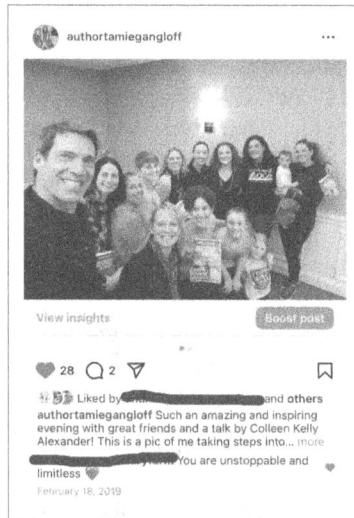

West Chester Women's Multisport LLC Book Signing with Colleen and her husband Sean, February 18, 2019.

Children with Chronic Medical Conditions and Pediatric Medical Traumatic Stress Could Lead to Eating Disorders and Body Image Issues

Colleen's profile and my own personal story touch on dealing with medical trauma and PTSD as an adult. Let's not forget that children and adolescents also encounter chronic illness and disturbed body image because of medical trauma and PTSD. In Chapter 1, I mentioned how broken and defective I felt following my scoliosis diagnosis as an adolescent. It's important for clinicians to recognize these potential mental health conditions when treating children and adolescents.

Pediatric-onset chronic illnesses impact up to 40 percent of school-aged children and adolescents in the U.S. (Pavilonis, n.d.). These illnesses, defined as medical conditions diagnosed in patients under 21 years of age and expected to last one year or more, are associated with mental health disorders and poor psychosocial functioning. Children impacted by chronic illness are specifically at risk for *pediatric medical traumatic stress* (PMTS). PMTS has been associated with problematic outcomes, including decreased adherence to medical treatments, and poorer quality of life (Cuneo et al., 2023, 2024).

In Chapter 4, I discussed Erik Erikson's stages of development and highlighted the impact of negative experiences and narratives, and how they become the messages individuals believe about themselves. Erikson describes each phase of development as the resolution of a psychosocial crisis, either positively or negatively (Anderson, 2016). *Psychosocial functioning* is defined as emotional, psychological, and social well-being and quality of life. In children and adolescents, personality is forming, so if psychosocial functioning is altered by illness, it can lead to mental health issues, including disordered eating.

Kiah's Story: Rheumatoid Arthritis, Anxiety, and Body Dysmorphia

Kiah is a 25-year-old woman living in Pennsylvania, whom I interviewed to discuss her challenges with chronic illness, mental health, and body image.

Some of Kiah's first memories are of going to doctor's appointments in preschool as she was diagnosed with rheumatoid arthritis (RA) when she was only two or three years old. RA is a chronic condition that affects the joints as well as other parts of the body. This did not hold her back from falling in love with dance at the age of five; she doesn't recall having any pain at that time. Several years later, she began to experience physical suffering and pain that she could not describe, and she returned to the rheumatologist. She recalls that her knees and feet started to ache, and it was unbearable at times.

At 12, she had to give up dance, the first passion of her life, due to her pain and limitations. Her parents sat her down and explained that she had something that was chronic, but she didn't fully grasp that concept at the time. Instead, she instantly felt loneliness by losing dance and her friends, community, and social interaction at the dance studio. She was isolated and started to experience depression at that time.

By the age of 15, Kiah was very thin and started to have flares of irritable bowel syndrome. She recalls being nauseous and having bad diarrhea within ten minutes of eating. She developed a fear of eating because she knew what the outcome was. Anytime she ate, she would feel so sick that she became averse to eating. She didn't have a desire to be thin or to lose weight, yet she had no craving for food or eating.

Kiah began to start the cycle of going to numerous doctor's appointments, only to be met with disappointment and no answers. Doctors attempted to treat her symptoms but found no cause. She slipped further into depression and tried different diets to try to feel better, to feel "normal." She was not able to find any solutions and "just dealt with it."

As a young adult, Kiah was in a long-term relationship that was unhealthy, which she later realized was a narcissistic relationship. This relationship, though she did not identify it with her symptoms at the time, caused her a great deal of anxiety, which caused her to lose a significant amount of weight because she could not eat or sleep. Kiah tried several different medications for anxiety and then gained weight due to an anti-anxiety medication. The weight gain worsened her RA symptoms and her intolerance to movement, including walking and household chores that involved bending, such as laundry or emptying the dishwasher. She became inactive due to her pain.

At that time, she was also in a fast-paced job, so she would skip breakfast in order not to get sick at work. She even got to the point of skipping lunch so she didn't risk having to run to the bathroom at work. She existed on a diet of coffee, water, and Goldfish crackers, as these were the things she could consume without getting sick. She also smoked cigarettes. She would wait to eat at home where she could be sick in peace. None of this behavior helped her chronic illness symptoms or her body image.

Kiah finally gained the courage to leave her abusive relationship and wanted to get help for her anxiety and other health symptoms. At this point, her physical illness worsened, and she lost a significant amount of weight in a short period of time. The noticeable weight loss was a wake-up call for Kiah and her family. She sat down with her parents and told them that she needed help, but she wanted to be at home with her dogs and did not want to go away to treatment. They obliged and helped her find medical resources. She met with her therapist and discussed treatment options and taking time off of work to go to treatment. She then entered treatment at a mental health partial hospitalization program and was treated for generalized anxiety as well as depression. During this treatment, she received a diagnosis of PTSD, and this was a game changer for her. It all finally made sense. She and her treatment team were able to refocus their work to process the trauma of her chronic illness and her abusive relationship.

Kiah received a new treatment for the condition, but these medications were not effective in managing her pain and symptoms. She began to have knee swelling for no reason, and she would have to have the fluid drained multiple times. She developed bursitis in her hips; her pain was so intense that she would limp to the car, and grocery shopping was very painful. She also began to experience pain in her sacroiliac joint, and she experienced "the most pain in the most places" compared to what she had ever experienced. Clearly, the medication she was taking for her RA was not working effectively.

Her doctor changed her medication, and it was life-giving. Today, Kiah is in much less pain. However, there are tradeoffs to taking it. This medication does make her immunocompromised, and she gets sick often. Colds last a long time, and cuts and scrapes linger and take a long time to heal. However, she is now in a routine that her body does not protest. She can now walk her dogs, do her laundry, and go to the gym.

Despite her PTSD and anxiety treatments and RA medication, Kiah still struggles with body image. She still wears clothes that are baggy. Due to the fluctuations in weight, she feels like she is in a body that is much larger than it is; however, when she looks in the mirror, she knows that this is not true. "I am learning to be okay with that, I physically see that."

Kiah understands the complexities of managing chronic illness, an eating disorder, and mental health challenges. She believes that it is a decision for her to keep up with her physical and mental health. In terms of her conditions, she believes "they are tapping you on the shoulder," and you have to choose not to listen to them and be unapologetic to yourself.

Erikson's Stages of Development and the Potential Impact of Chronic Illness on Disordered Eating and Diminished Body Image

Body image issues, eating disorders, and chronic illness may impact children and adolescents differently depending on their specific age and circumstances and the medical events that they have encountered. Even without chronic illness and potential trauma surrounding it, each of Erikson's stages includes a psychosocial crisis. An individual either ends up in the positive or negative spectrum of this crisis, based on the events of this phase and how it was handled by their caregivers (Anderson, 2016). While there is a lot of grey on the spectrum, a child or adolescent will tend to be on one side of the line when they leave each stage of development.

Here is how a child or adolescent may experience medical trauma associated with a chronic illness in each stage of development:

Infancy: Trust vs. Mistrust

Love, holding, and bonding during infancy are essential. This can be disrupted if there is a medical condition that becomes chronic. Medical treatments and hospital stays may keep an infant from physical touch which is essential in this phase of development. In infancy, we develop basic trust and that is embedded in our psyche. Basic trust comes from needs being met by a caregiver. Mistrust in this phase of development continues to carry throughout the lifespan.

Toddler: Autonomy vs. Shame and Doubt

Toddlers want to learn and ask how and try to do everything on their own. They want to master certain tasks. What if they are not capable of doing these tasks such as learning to tie their shoes as a result of physical limitations? They can end up in shame and doubt. Caregivers may ask what they can do if their child has such physical limitations.

Preschool: Initiative vs. Guilt

Children at this age want to do everything and help caregivers with tasks. They see Dad making dinner or Mom vacuuming, and they want to do it as well. Guilt comes from not feeling like they are taking initiative, and they end up feeling guilty because of the things they couldn't do. They may be aware of their limitations from a chronic illness, and it could impact their sense of self at this stage.

School Age: Industry vs. Inferiority

At this stage, kids really start to explore the world and try new things such as sports and music lessons. If they can't do the things they want to or try including the things their peers are able to do, they can end up feeling inferior. The drive to compare starts to show up in this stage of development. This is where kids start to notice that they are different from their peers and where we start to see concrete body image concerns. Body image distress, related to illness, can be a factor that leads to an eating disorder.

Adolescence: Identity vs. Confusion

This stage can be summed up with the question "Who am I?" Adolescents are trying to figure out who they are and their identity. If identity formation is disrupted by chronic illness, clinicians and loved ones see identity confusion and ruptures in self. This is also the stage where individuals develop their sense of self, including body image.

All Stages Can Lead to Body Image Issues and Disordered Eating

When analyzing the stages of development, an individual's sense of self, security, and abilities are all tied together. Ruptures during any of these phases, let alone all of them, will likely lead to mental health concerns including anxiety, depression, PTSD, and disordered eating. Experiencing feelings that their body is failing may intensify body hatred in children and adolescents, increasing body dissatisfaction and eating disorder symptoms.

The impact of these ruptures can last throughout the lifespan, unless individuals are able to address it. If the rupture occurred during infancy, a clinician needs to focus on the mistrust that may have resulted. Reflecting on my personal experience, I wore a body cast as a newborn, as the result of hip dysplasia. This prevented my parents from being able to bond fully as the cast interrupted that. Attachment ruptures of this kind are lasting and can impact relationships throughout an individual's life. Fast-forward a decade, I experienced obstacles as an adolescent because of my scoliosis. At this phase, I knew that I didn't fit in. I was skinny, I wore a back brace, and I was made fun of for being a nerd (one of the smart kids). I had a poor sense of self and distorted body image in part because of my chronic illness and the medical procedures required to treat it.

A psychosocial crisis at any stage will cause a disruption of self. If this occurs at all stages, there is hope! While clinicians know that they don't need to help a client "dig up" everything from the past, if they see the impacts from that stage of development in a client, clinicians need to address that.

Suggestions for Clinicians to Screen for Medical Trauma and PTSD

There are several screenings available for clinicians and other medical providers to use with clients who may have experienced medical trauma or have PTSD. Here are a few recommendations.

For primary care physicians, the *Primary Care PTSD Screen for DSM-5* (PC-PTSD-5) is recommended. A physician starts with asking if their patient has experienced a traumatic event in their life (sexual assault, a serious accident, a war, etc.). If the answer is yes, the questionnaire is administered. This is a five-question survey of yes or no questions inquiring about nightmares, hypervigilance, feelings of guilt and shame. Yes answers then require further investigation (Prins et al., 2022).

The *Trauma Screen Questionnaire (TSF)* is a ten-question self-report survey that can be administered in a primary care or mental health setting. It assesses the client's experiences over the past two weeks to assess for a stress response to a traumatic event. This survey also includes questions related to hypervigilance, visceral reactions, and intrusive thoughts (Brewin, 2014).

For mental health providers, the *PTSD Checklist for DSM-5* (PCL-5) is a 20-question survey to determine a PTSD diagnosis as well as periodically repeating it throughout the treatment process as a means of tracking progress. The questionnaire includes questions related to unwanted memories or dreams, visceral reactions to memories, irritability, difficulty concentrating, and so forth. This should be administered and evaluated by a clinician (Weathers et al., 2013).

Exercises for Clinicians to Use to Uncover Potential Trauma and Stress

The following exercises can help your clients work through their journey with chronic illness. These can help you address underlying topics with your clients and may uncover past trauma and stress that may be helpful in a client's eating disorder treatment.

Exercise 8.1: Survey Your Client's Journey

Start by gathering more information about the history of a client's illness during each phase of development. I would start by including these questions:

1   When were you first diagnosed with your illness?
2   Do you have a memory of that diagnosis? Be as specific as possible: How did you receive the news? How did your parents/family react?
3   If you do not have a memory, what have you been told about that time in your life? How were you treated? Were you hospitalized for periods of time?
4   What were you thinking and feeling at that time?
5   Did you notice an increase in anxiety after your diagnosis?
6   Did you struggle with intrusive thoughts about your illness?
7   Do you have a fear of medical providers or medical settings as a result of your illness?
8   Did you notice thoughts about your body at that time?
9   At what point did you notice that you had some negative thoughts about your body, whether that was related to appearance or function?
10   Have you ever felt like you "left your body" to avoid experiencing what was happening to you? Some describe it as a feeling of floating above their body.

Exercise 8.2: Make a Lifemap with Clients

Some treatment providers have their clients complete a lifemap or a timeline of all of the significant events that have occurred in their lives. Oftentimes, illness may be an afterthought and may not receive a mention on the life map. If there is a known illness, I would ask your client to complete this lifemap to include significant events, both positive and negative. This should include anything impactful and document illness, surgery, and medical procedures, in addition to other life events as well as other mental health concerns, such as the lifespan of their eating disorder.

If your client doesn't have a memory related to these topics, remind them that their diagnosis may have been related to something preverbal, but that doesn't mean that it didn't have a big impact. You are developing trust and mistrust during that earliest phase of development that could become more significant with development.

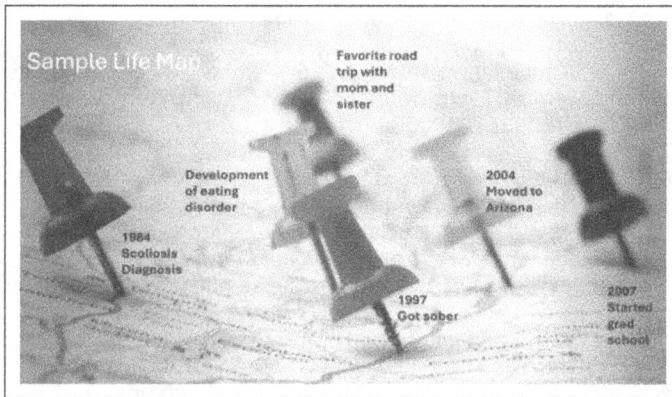

Sample life map (based on my own experience)

Summary

The psychosocial stages of development shed some light on the impact of chronic illness diagnosed in childhood and how this can impact patients throughout their lifespan. Medical trauma can occur in a number of healthcare settings and can lead to medical traumatic stress or PTSD. There are several recommended screening tools that clinicians can use to assess and then plan treatment for those impacted. We learned from lived experiences in this chapter to demonstrate the impact of chronic illness in an individual's life and how it may alter someone's body image and coping mechanisms. The next section of this book will push more into how chronic illness and the medical system can impact self-care and body image, leading to disordered eating.

References

Alexander, C. K. (2018). *Gratitude in Motion*. Center Street.
American Psychological Association. (2020). PTSD Treatment: Information for Patients and Families. www.apa.org/ptsd-guideline/patients-and-families
Anderson, K. (2016, February 5). Kathy Anderson's Psychology Channel: Erikson's Theory of Psychosocial Development. YouTube. https://youtu.be/z1c1y-mm_io?si=gb4ykVZUmTyUjdEC

Brewin. (2014). Trauma Screening Questionnaire (TSQ). U.S. Department of Veterans Affairs. www.ptsd.va.gov/professional/assessment/screens/tsq.asp

Cuneo, A., Sifflet, C., Bardach, N., Ly, N., von Scheven, E., & Perito, E. R. (2023). Pediatric medical traumatic stress and trauma-informed care in pediatric chronic illness: A healthcare provider survey. *The Journal of Pediatrics, 261*, 113580. https://doi.org/10.1016/j.jpeds.2023.113580

Cuneo, A., Smith-Thomas, T., & Marsac, M. (2024). Opportunities for trauma-informed medical care in cystic fibrosis. *Pediatric Pulmonology, 59*(6), 1814–1816. https://doi.org/10.1002/ppul.26962

Oregon Health & Science University. (2012, September 28). One-fifth of spine surgery patients develop PTSD symptoms. *ScienceDaily*. www.sciencedaily.com/releases/2012/09/120928103800.htm

Pavilonis, V. (n.d.). Fact check: More than 40% of children have chronic illness, CDC says. USA TODAY. www.usatoday.com/story/news/factcheck/2022/02/10/fact-check-more-than-40-children-have-chronic-illness-cdc-says/6639320001

Prins, A., Bovin, M. J., Kimerling, R , Kaloupek, D. G, Marx, B. P., Pless Kaiser, A., & Schnurr, P. P. (2015). *Primary Care PTSD Screen for DSM-5 (PC-PTSD-5)* [Measurement instrument]. www.ptsd.va.gov/professional/assessment/documents/pc-ptsd5-screen.pdf

Weathers, F. W., Litz, B. T., Keane, T. M., Palmieri, P. A., Marx, B. P., & Schnurr, P. P. (2013). The PTSD Checklist for DSM-5 (PCL-5) – Standard [Measurement instrument]. www.ptsd.va.gov/professional/assessment/documents/PCL5_Standard_form_week.PDF

Part 4

Managing and Treating Chronic Illness and Eating Disorders

Part 4 focuses on the treatment of individuals with chronic medical conditions and eating disorders. I will define weight stigma in the medical field and discuss its implications, including how it can predispose individuals to disordered eating. A significant emphasis will be placed on minimizing the impact of weighing patients in medical settings.

I will review recommended treatment modalities and suggested activities for clinicians. These modalities will include narrative therapy, EMDR, and acceptance and commitment therapy, among others. This section will also explore the therapeutic alliance within medical treatment teams, the role of physical therapists, and strategies to bridge the gap between different disciplines.

Additionally, I will discuss the psychology of sports injuries and how it can benefit individuals with chronic illnesses and eating disorders. You will hear my story of a sports injury, as well as that of Hope.

Each chapter will include relevant research findings and conclude with practical suggestions for clinicians. I will also highlight moments from my own life that pertain to the chapter topics.

- Chapter 9: Navigating Weight Stigma, Health System Pressures, and Self-Care Amid Chronic Illness and Eating Disorders
- Chapter 10: Recommended Treatment Modalities
- Chapter 11: From Specialists to Support: Key Steps in Finding the Ideal Medical Team
- Chapter 12: Sports Injury Versus Chronic Medical Condition—What's the Difference?

DOI: 10.4324/9781003500254-12

Navigating Weight Stigma, Health System Pressures, and Self-Care Amid Chronic Illness and Eating Disorders

The Dangerous Focus on Weight Management in Those with Chronic Illnesses

Weight stigma in medicine creates a perfect storm to cause an eating disorder or lead to a relapse with an eating disorder in those with chronic illness. Many people living with chronic illnesses see medical providers frequently and may undergo medical procedures regularly, making them vulnerable to an overfocus on their weight. This chapter looks at how the healthcare system overemphasizes weight and offers suggestions to clinicians and medical practitioners about how to navigate this problematic position in medicine today.

What Is Weight Stigma in Medicine?

Weight stigma, also known as *weight bias*, refers to beliefs, attitudes, negativity, and discrimination based solely on someone's weight or size. This generally targets people who are in larger bodies, but it can impact anyone of any size (Edwards-Gayfield, n.d.).

Although doctors typically do not intend to show weight bias, this can occur both explicitly and implicitly through *microaggressions*. Microaggression is a term that encompasses both verbal and nonverbal behaviors against people in marginalized or non-mainstream groups. According to the Cleveland Clinic (2022):

> Microaggression was first used around 1970 by Harvard psychiatrist Dr. Chester Pierce. Dr. Pierce used this term to describe the regular insults and dismissals he witnessed people who were non-Black using against people who were Black. He believed these experiences could have a major impact on a person's psychological and physical health over time.

Research demonstrates that providers communicate less effectively with individuals from stigmatized racial groups and those facing weight-related

DOI: 10.4324/9781003500254-13

stigma. These negative provider attitudes contribute to disparities in care. Studies show that implicit biases are linked to lower patient satisfaction ratings. When combined, implicit and explicit negative attitudes toward those in larger bodies create obstacles to patient-centered communication. Implicit (unconscious) and explicit (conscious) biases are both defined as attitudes or stereotypes that affect understanding, actions, and decisions in an unconscious manner. This, in turn, increases the risk of nonadherence to medical recommendations by 19 percent, fostering mistrust and leading to poorer wellness outcomes, recovery, and mental health. Addressing these biases is crucial for improving patient care and health outcomes for marginalized groups (Phelan et al., 2015).

Does Weight Stigma Lead to Disordered Eating?

There are studies that discuss the connection between disordered eating and weight stigma. Here are a few that link negative attitudes about weight to problematic outcomes for individuals.

In the field of eating disorder medicine, clinicians typically avoid using the term *obesity*, which medically refers to individuals with a *body mass index* (BMI) over 30. Obesity is often strongly stigmatized and associated with negative perceptions. Research indicates that individuals with obesity often trigger feelings of disgust, anger, blame, and dislike in others. Despite the fact that nearly one-third of the adult population in the United States is classified as obese, individuals in this group frequently face prejudice, derogatory comments, and inadequate treatment across various settings, including healthcare. Additionally, there is increasing evidence that healthcare professionals, including physicians, tend to harbor strong negative views toward people with obesity (Phelan et al., 2015).

One of the biggest risks for developing an eating disorder is having a history of dieting and attempts to lose weight. When medical providers encourage patients to lose weight, it can lead to unhealthy behaviors such as restriction, excessive exercise, and purging. A strong emphasis on BMI often hinders doctors from properly assessing for eating disorders. In fact, individuals with a higher BMI are more likely to meet the criteria for an eating disorder (Westby et al., 2021).

Prior to recommending weight loss, doctors should assess for eating disorders and be careful when recommending weight loss for health or as a surgical requirement. Weight stigma in medicine is harmful and can prevent someone from getting needed medical care. Patients may develop a fear of going to the doctor as they have experienced discrimination and invalidation.

Risks of Presurgical Weight Loss Recommendations

Historically, medical providers have recommended or required weight loss prior to surgeries such as knee and hip replacements. This recommendation is known to cause disordered eating. We know the basics: weight loss is caused by strategic caloric intake, overall wellness, and activity. If you are in the market for a new knee or hip, my guess is that it isn't because you are running or riding your bike carefree with no pain! Prescribing weight loss almost calls for someone to engage in disordered behavior as they may not be able to increase movement. The other option is caloric restriction and potentially exercising through immense pain. Obviously, this is a simplistic view, but it is also an accurate representation.

I have seen many friends struggle with this, especially those with chronic illnesses. They have had years of challenges with weight loss, pain, surgery, more pain, and more struggle. I have had reports from physical therapists that their patients have disclosed the use of eating-disordered behaviors to lose weight for surgery only to find that the disordered behavior continued after surgery and recovery. We already know that surgery causes changes in appetite and that we need more energy and protein post-op. So, these patients are going into surgery with a nutritional deficiency that will then inhibit healing. With the mindset that weight loss equals health, some patients may continue this behavior until developing a diagnosed eating disorder.

Newer studies are showing that presurgical weight loss is contraindicated. We now have some solid evidence that presurgical weight loss causes more complications and increased risk of postsurgical infections. A study by Inacio and colleagues (2014) evaluated patients who lost weight prior to a knee or hip replacement surgery and kept the weight off postoperatively. Their findings showed a higher rate of postoperative deep surgical site infection and a higher rate of readmission. This discovery brings into question the safety of weight management before total replacement of the hip and knee joints. Further research is needed to determine the safety of weight management before total replacement (Inacio et al., 2014). Additionally, there is limited evidence to support the recommendation of weight loss in the year prior to total joint arthroplasty and to determine the effectiveness of short-term non-pharmacological, non-surgical weight management interventions on patient and surgical outcomes, according to Lui et al. (2015).

Lived Experiences with Weight Management and Chronic Illness During Surgery

Let me tell you two different stories about how this dangerous focus on weight management impacted my own medical treatment for scoliosis.

These stories can provide a clinician with a perspective on the challenges of chronic illnesses and eating disorders, which should give some insight into how to assist with eating disorder treatment.

As I stated long ago in Chapter 1, my first spine surgery was in my 20s when I was still very much in my eating disorder. For many spine surgeries, an important component is physical therapy, sometimes pre-op and most often post-op. I recall my physical therapist also asking me if I had eaten before coming to my appointments. I would often show up with a cup of Wawa coffee and I often told the truth, that I had "not eaten yet" that day. I was not thinking about what my body needed to heal because I was stuck in my eating disorder symptoms.

This situation was not just problematic for everyday living, but it was slowing my healing from surgery because bodies need a lot of energy to heal. Not only was I not giving myself enough energy, I was going without adequate protein or rest. Combine this with another bad habit I had: smoking. I was not willing to give it up either; I only did so for about two weeks—one week prior to surgery and one week after when I kindly threatened my roommate to give me a cigarette. I already knew that smoking was bad for bone health, though my self-destructive tendencies did not seem to care about that.

Over time, I recovered from surgery and was able to return to work, but I was not strong and did not continue to do my physical therapy exercises. My focus turned to my weight and attempting to exercise, emphasizing weight loss instead of healing and getting stronger. I was not yet recovered from my eating disorder and was still entrenched in eating disorder thoughts and behaviors. Because of my eating disorder, I was not able to heal from my spine surgery in an efficient or healthy way.

Many years later, prior to the big surgery on my spine, I dealt with weight concerns, even though I had been recovered from my eating disorder for many years. (For my purposes, I am using the term *recovered*; however, you can use whatever works for you as we know that recovery is a spectrum.) This happened because I was in several scoliosis and chronic illness Facebook groups where many were commiserating and telling horror stories (I did remove myself from these groups eventually—I needed only positivity leading into that surgery). One of the common topics was that you should lose ten pounds before surgery. This stunned me and led me to question the reasons behind this topic. *Why? Is there a medical reason for this?* My doctor didn't mention weight loss at all, so I ignored this. However, the vascular surgeon did need to "lay eyes on me" to make sure I wasn't "too big" to gain access to my spine through my abdomen, language that appalled me.

After this experience, I instantly felt angry and empathy for those experiencing weight bias in the medical system. There are so many people who are denied surgery due to their weight, being told to lose weight before they are eligible. This can cause someone to *not* get the necessary treatment and lead to disordered eating in someone who didn't have a prior eating disorder.

Others who I have worked with have also documented harmful comments from their doctors regarding their weight, chronic illness, and management strategies. For example, after a recent conference talk, a woman came up to me and stated that she was diagnosed with scoliosis as a kid and was braced. She was so uncomfortable in the brace as it was not something she could hide under clothing, and doctors could not mold it to fit her shape. She was in a larger body, and she stated that she always had been, even as a kid. Her doctor told her that her scoliosis would correct itself if she lost weight.

This is so far from the truth! It is such an awful thing to say to anyone, as if she was being blamed for her scoliosis. She did not disclose if she had her own personal eating disorder history, yet I can imagine that this history could lead to body image distress. She said that it led to depression and isolation as she did not want to wear her brace. To this day, her curve has not progressed, even though she did not lose the prescribed weight.

The fact that this doctor said this to her is not only egregious but flat-out wrong and shows the inherent biases against larger bodies in the medical system. There is no connection to larger bodies and scoliosis: the average BMI of someone with scoliosis is in the lower range, which could be due to many factors, including the difficulty with eating while wearing a back brace, as it is tight around the stomach, similar to a corset. Comments about weight can lead to lasting body image concerns and contribute to the development of an eating disorder.

Steps to Combat the Overfocus on Weight in Medicine for Those with Chronic Illnesses

"Please Don't Weigh Me Unless It's Medically Necessary"

There is a new movement within healthcare systems to decline to step on the scale to avoid weight bias from doctors. This can be a positive step forward for those who have eating disorder symptoms and those who do not want to be judged by their weight in the medical system. Research shows that over half of individuals, when asked to be weighed at medical appointments, felt it negatively impacted their mental health and raised concerns about potential weight-based discrimination. Notably, being weighed is often found to be medically unnecessary. This has led to a significant trend, with 30 percent of women now refusing to be weighed and some even avoiding healthcare settings altogether to avoid the scale (McCuien, 2023).

If a patient has an eating disorder and chronic illness, they run the risk of being weighed often. They may not feel that they can say no to this, and their eating-disordered self may want to see the number. The eating disorder can use that number as ammunition to fuel disordered behaviors. "My weight was higher today, so I have to restrict." "My weight was lower—I'm doing a good job and I have to continue." "My weight was the same—I'm not trying hard enough." The eating disorder thoughts are ruthless, and knowledge of weight can only serve to increase these thoughts.

Additionally, most scales are calibrated differently, and often the number is inconsistent on different scales. Recently, I was weighed twice, within a week, at two different medical offices, and my weight was vastly different. While I know that body weight fluctuates daily, based on many factors, it typically does not vary *that* much. I thought it was a little ridiculous. Gosh, if I had been in an active eating disorder, this could have sent me down a spiral of body image panic and symptom use.

My Personal Experience

After a busy month of travel, I ended up in urgent care with bronchitis. Nurses checked my weight, which seems ridiculous. What does my weight have to do with bronchitis?! When the doctor came in, I brought it up to him—I wouldn't be me if I didn't. I told him that if I was XX pounds heavier or had a higher BMI, they would probably have prescribed weight loss in addition to my Z-pack. He did laugh, but I was happy that he agreed with my sentiment. My goal was to make the point that there is no need to weigh someone because of a cough.

Many people have a couple of medical appointments each year: maybe an annual physical, an annual gynecology visit for those with female parts, and a sick visit. If an individual has an injury or chronic medical condition, the number of medical appointments they have increases exponentially. I cannot tell you how many I have had in the past year. If I include physical therapy visits, that number increases by about 40. Good thing physical therapists don't weigh us.

Often providers require a weight when an individual arrives at their appointment. They may find this simply annoying, but it could trigger more harmful thoughts. Sometimes I say no, and if they are insistent, I will explain why they shouldn't require a weigh-in. I have even offered to provide staff training, given my professional experience. For many, *if* a weight is deemed medically necessary, a blind weigh-in is best.

Should We Do Weight Exposures?

There is limited research on whether *blind weights* (where a patient is not informed of their weight) or *open weighing* (where a patient is told their weight) leads to better patient outcomes. Clinician preference is roughly split 50/50 between the two methods. Many clinicians decide whether to use blind or open weighing based on the client's presentation, comorbid issues, and the rationale behind allowing patients to see their weight or not.

Research indicates that clients who have recovered from eating disorders experience varying levels of anxiety regarding weight visibility, often influenced by their previous treatment experiences, as reported in a study by Froreich et al. (2020). Blind weights can increase anxiety due to the uncertainty of not knowing the number, while seeing the weight can act as a reality check. However, some patients reported feelings of losing autonomy or feeling punished when informed of their weight. Others experienced reduced anxiety when they did not have to see the number, describing it as "one less thing to worry about," or feeling that they were not yet ready to confront the scale. Once trust was established in their treatment team, many clients felt comfortable with not knowing their weight. The study concluded that most patients preferred blind weighing over open weighing.

In treatment centers, there are times when it is clinically appropriate for clinicians to do weight exposures. This means that a clinician would have a client step on the scale to see their weight. This is very client specific and determined on a case-by-case basis. For example, a client may be returning to a college sport that has a weight requirement. It would be appropriate to do this exposure in treatment to have a chance to process it. Occasionally, an outpatient dietitian may do these exposures with a client who might benefit from a "reality check." This can also be tricky and is up to the judgment of an experienced eating disorder specialist. Sometimes, a client benefits from seeing the actual number to show that their weight hasn't changed dramatically or to know the accurate number.

For a client with a chronic medical condition, I believe it may be appropriate for them to engage in weight exposures with their dietitian, depending on their recovery stage. This approach is particularly important if the client's medical condition requires regular weight checks for medical reasons. In such cases, using blind weights, advocating for less frequent weight checks, and allowing the client to see the number on the scale can all be beneficial. When suitable, clinicians will incorporate weight exposures to help the client become comfortable with seeing the number on the scale. This approach can be especially useful for someone returning to sports or managing a medical condition that necessitates weight monitoring.

Recommendations for Primary Care Physicians

Medical providers should consider recommendations so that patients with larger bodies feel more comfortable and accepted. The medical system can also start with less focus on weight and not ask for patient weights at each visit. If there are medical concerns or potential risks for obesity-related disease, the focus should be on wellness and preventative measures that do not focus on weight or require getting on the scale. Phelan et al. (2015) recommend further research in this area. A patient–doctor relationship should be one with mutual trust and collaboration and not feel punitive in any way. We will discuss this further in Chapter 11.

Suggestions for Clinicians

There are a few approaches clinicians can use to help their clients navigate chronic illness with body image issues. I have included instructions as well as exercises for clinicians to use to assist individuals with chronic illnesses and eating disorders to manage the emphasis on weight within the medical system.

Our Bodies Need a Lot of Energy to Heal

Surgery or illness is not the time to focus on weight loss. When people are immobilized, they often worry about gaining weight. It's important for an individual not to decrease their caloric intake just because they are inactive. In fact, their calorie needs may be greater than usual during this time, as their body requires energy and protein to support the healing process. Meeting their overall energy and protein needs is crucial to prevent the breakdown of body tissues such as muscles and ligaments. This will help ensure a smooth healing process and promote a quicker recovery (Hospital for Special Surgery, 2009). "Poor nutrition before or during the healing process can delay [an individual's] healing," says registered dietitian Kavitha Krishnan, RD. "While eating well can help the body heal faster and fight infection" (Cleveland Clinic, 2023).

Exercises for Clinicians

What can we do as clinicians? Here are a few ideas:

- We distribute those lovely cards "Please don't weigh me unless it's medically necessary" or letters of support for our clients to use with their medical providers.
- We work on empowering our clients not only to use these tools but also to use their voices, which I believe is even more important than the cards or letters.
- We talk through what being weighed at a medical office brings up for clients. Some medical offices ask if individuals want to be weighed; however, this is not the norm. If a clinician is treating a client with a chronic illness, talk to them about their experience with being weighed at their medical appointments.

Exercise 9.1: Role Play with Your Client

Do some role-playing and practice with a client what to say when a medical assistant is insistent on getting that number into the chart. Also, consider how common it is for an individual to get a blind weight only to have their weight listed on the after-visit summary, and talk this out with the client.

If clinicians are not practicing this with their clients, they are missing a potentially significant trigger. In treatment, clinicians do exposures at the grocery store or clothing store. Let's do exposures and practice what it is like to go to the doctor's office and advocate and say "no thank you" when asked to step on the scale. A client might get a strong reaction when they are asked to slip off those shoes and step on the scale. Practicing handling these reactions is just as important as it is to practice asking family members not to make body comments!

Exercise 9.2: Encourage the Use of a Registered Dietitian

There are many recommendations regarding caloric intake as well as the types of foods that will assist in healing that can help a client. A dietitian is a client's ally in planning ahead. A client doesn't only want to plan ahead for a scheduled surgery, but they want to have a plan in place for when an injury or surgery may occur. With chronic illness, it is not "if" someone will have a setback or surgical needs, it is "when." Planning ahead, just as we plan for a pain flare, will make sure a client is prepared and will decrease anxiety, fear of the unknown, and the likelihood of a potential relapse with eating disorder symptoms.

Talk to your client about the benefits of using a registered dietitian because they:

- Can help meal plan/prepare ahead of time for potential surgery/illness setback
- Can help prepare for weight exposures in a medical setting
- Can consider how a client can be prepared for nourishment during surgery and injury recovery/flares

Exercise 9.3: Steps a Clinician or Registered Dietitian Can Take with Clients to Prepare for a Medical Procedure or a Flare

- Create a postsurgical meal plan. Nausea and loss of appetite are normal postoperatively and may last a lengthy time depending on the surgery. Help your client plan ahead for meals that are nourishing as well as easy to access/prepare.
- Ensure that a client will have adequate nutrition in the hospital. Their doctor can order supplements, as they may not be able to eat enough calories for healing.
- Discuss a meal plan for when a client experiences a pain flare or setback. This might be similar to a postsurgical meal plan. Your client should always have foods at home that are easy to access in case they are having a setback. Setbacks are, of course, always unplanned.

- Work with a client on weight exposure in sessions.
- Empower the client to advocate for themselves and utilize a no-weigh card.
- Reach out to your client's medical providers to discuss whether blind or open weigh-ins are appropriate when they are in their eating disorder recovery.

Summary

In our medical system, weight stigma exists and can lead to noncompliance with medical recommendations, avoidance of medical appointments, or denial or lack of necessary care. Weight bias in medicine can lead to disordered eating or to a relapse in those with an existing eating disorder history. Newer studies show that presurgical weight loss is contraindicated and may cause harm. There is a need for further research on weight exposures; however, someone with a chronic illness is faced with the scale at many medical appointments, so we need to prepare our clients. Bodies require energy and rest to heal. A dietitian is a client's partner in creating a meal plan that works for times of illness, wellness, and surgery. The next chapter will focus on treatment modalities.

References

Cleveland Clinic. (2022, February 2). What are microaggressions? https://health. clevelandclinic.org/what-are-microaggressions-and-examples

Cleveland Clinic. (2023, January 31). What to eat when you're trying to heal. https:// health.clevelandclinic.org/foods-to-help-healing

Edwards-Gayfield, P. (n.d.). What is weight stigma? National Eating Disorders Association. www.nationaleatingdisorders.org/weight-stigma

Froreich, F. V., Ratcliffe, S. E., & Vartanian, L. R. (2020). Blind versus open weighing from an eating disorder patient perspective. *Journal of Eating Disorders*, *8*(39). https://doi.org/10.1186/s40337-020-00316-1

Hospital for Special Surgery. (2009). Nutrition for healing after surgery. www.hss. edu/conditions_nutrition-for-healing.asp

Inacio, M. C. S., Kritz-Silverstein, D., Raman, R., Macera, C. A., Nichols, J. F., Shaffer, R. A., & Fithian, D. C. (2014). The risk of surgical site infection and re-admission in obese patients undergoing total joint replacement who lose weight before surgery and keep it off post-operatively. *The Bone & Joint Journal*, *96-B*(5), 629–635. https://doi.org/10.1302/0301-620x.96b5.33136

Lui, M., Jones, C. A., & Westby, M. D. (2015). Effect of non-surgical, non-pharmacological weight loss interventions in patients who are obese prior to hip and knee arthroplasty surgery: A rapid review. *Systematic Reviews*, *4*(1), 121. https://doi. org/10.1186/s13643-015-0107-2

McCuien, P. (2023, July 25). Study shows that weighing female patients at health care visits is associated with negative mental health. Medical Xpress. https:// medicalxpress.com/news/2023-07-female-patients-health-negative-mental.html

Phelan, S. M., Burgess, D. J., Yeazel, M. W., Hellerstedt, W. L., Griffin, J. M., & van Ryn, M. (2015). Impact of weight bias and stigma on quality of care and outcomes for patients with obesity. *Obesity Reviews, 16*(4), 319–326. https://doi. org/10.1111/obr.12266

Westby, A., Jones, C. M., & Loth, K. A. (2021). The role of weight stigma in the development of eating disorders. *American Family Physician, 104*(1), 7–9. www. aafp.org/pubs/afp/issues/2021/0700/p7.html

Chapter 10

Recommended Treatment Modalities

In previous chapters, I discussed trauma related to medical treatments and chronic illness. The next step in helping an individual heal from trauma associated with chronic illness and an eating disorder is to help them find the mental health treatments that work best for their specific needs. There are several types of therapy that may be beneficial for your clients, which I detail in this chapter. These include narrative therapy, play therapy, eye movement desensitization and reprocessing therapy, acceptance and commitment therapy, attachment therapy, and progressive desensitization.

Laying the Foundation for Trauma Work with Safety and Containment

We cannot do trauma work without establishing *safety* and *containment*. Safety means that we are helping our clients to commit to safety regarding not using self-harm or acting out using unhealthy coping skills. The work we have done with coping skills allows our clients to keep themselves safe. Another level of safety is emotional safety. As clinicians, we do this by establishing rapport and trust with our clients so they feel comfortable enough to be vulnerable and work through their trauma. It is essential for an individual to have a safe, calm place to heal. Clinicians must work with individuals to create a plan that emphasizes physical and emotional safety. Containment is the ability to create a safe mental space where we can gently place our painful memories and feelings, helping us to manage them more effectively. I detail strategies and exercises in this chapter that can help clients create safety and containment (such as Exercise 10.1 on creating a containment box and Exercise 10.2 on writing a narrative). Some of these strategies and tools are from my own days of treatment for an eating disorder, many years ago, when I began work on my trauma. The skills that I learned at that time are still helpful in my life today.

DOI: 10.4324/9781003500254-14

Types of Therapy for Chronic Illness and Eating Disorders

Narrative Therapy

First and foremost, *narrative therapy* allows an individual to externalize their problem so it is seen as separate from, not part of, themselves. Narrative therapy was developed in the 1980s by Michael White and David Epstom (Vinney, 2019). Narrative therapy embraces a compassionate approach by recognizing that the individual is the expert of their own experiences. It seeks to understand their story without labeling or blaming, fostering a supportive environment where they can explore and make sense of their life's challenges. This approach aims to break the problem into smaller bites (pun intended) so that it feels more manageable and less overwhelming. Individuals can then review the story they tell themselves about their identified problems and challenges. The goal is to create a healthy narrative.

An individual can begin narrative therapy by going back to some of my initial observations about living with a chronic illness—that individuals are in long-term relationships with their medical conditions (and can even bestow a name on them!). This perspective is the first step in changing the narrative. Living a life in a body that an individual did not "choose" can feel suffocating. If someone can change that message to say that they are in a committed relationship with their body, medical condition, and abilities, then they also have permission and the power to make changes. They are no longer sentenced to live in a body that they did not choose; they are in a body that they can partner with, support, love, give empathy to, show compassion for, challenge, and grow. In my life, Titanium isn't who I am; Titanium is my partner.

I get it—this may sound a little "out there" to some. A client may be thinking, "How on earth can you say that I can partner with this body?! I did not want this, I don't like how I look or feel, the pain I have, the challenges ahead of me." I get it, and I validate that. I have felt that way—I can still slip into those thoughts. However, they are only fleeting now. Today, I have this powerful vessel to live life. And yes, part of life means that I have extra rest days, setbacks, surgery, and challenges. I have been able to learn and grow from each experience. That is not to say that those experiences weren't rough and scary and agonizing at times. I have a level of resilience that is strong because I have had to work at it.

I would guess that many individuals could benefit from reframing their story by shifting it from their chronic illness *doing something to them* to instead *being in relationship* with their chronic illness. They have that power and strength. They are stronger than they can imagine and have the ability to partner with their illness; it is a part of who they are. It does not define them. They can choose to love this part of themselves just as they love their intelligence, hair, dimples, sense of style, or sense of humor.

To begin, help your clients start a journal and ask them what their narrative is. I will describe this in more detail in Exercise 10.2. Narrative therapy is an ongoing process and a skill that is learned over time. Once developed, this skill allows us to continue to reframe our thoughts and change the narrative throughout our lifespan. Narrative therapy can be time-limited, such as EMDR, if we are focusing on one specific narrative; focused treatment can take several months. Many clinicians utilize narrative therapy as one of the treatment modalities they use in their practice and it is often done in conjunction with other treatment modalities such as CBT and DBT.

Play Therapy

Play therapy is an evidence-based treatment that helps children express themselves through both directive and nondirective play. Since children often lack the verbal and processing skills to articulate their feelings, play provides a safe and natural way for them to communicate (Therapist.com, 2021). Play therapy is typically used for children under the age of 12; however, it can be helpful to use for adolescents or adults as well. It can be used to process issues including chronic illness, divorce, aggressive behavior, grief, and eating disorders (Pietrangelo, 2019).

Medical providers in pediatric hospitals know that medical procedures can be scary and painful for children. This can lead to feelings of trauma in their young patients (Locatelli, 2019). It can be assumed that some of these children will experience pediatric medical traumatic stress, discussed in more detail in Chapter 9. Medical traumatic stress can lead to PTSD. However, this is often overlooked in an outpatient setting. If a child presents for therapy with mood dysregulation, the assumption may be made that the focus is on interpersonal family systems, and we may not address the medical trauma. When a child and therapist build a strong, trusting relationship, and when the child feels supported with both structure and compassion, they can begin to work through their past traumas. In this safe and nurturing environment, children can regain their sense of security and learn to overcome their fears. As I mentioned in Chapter 8, sometimes children who go through traumatic medical experiences might feel detached from their primary caregivers.

Play therapists who work with young children in nonmedical settings should be mindful of the possibility of medical trauma, even if it is not immediately recognized as a presenting issue. A child's experiences with painful or scary medical procedures may come to light during assessments, particularly when gathering a comprehensive developmental and medical history. Additionally, clinicians should inform the child's parents and teachers about the links between medical trauma and the child's behavioral and emotional challenges (Locatelli, 2019).

Eye Movement Desensitization and Reprocessing Therapy

Eye movement desensitization and reprocessing (EMDR) *therapy* is an approach designed to help alleviate the psychological effects of trauma. In this process, clients engage in bilateral stimulation while processing their traumatic memories. Importantly, clients do not need to discuss the specifics of their trauma to work through it, and progress is often observed more quickly compared to traditional talk therapy (EMDR International Association, 2022).

When a therapist and client collaboratively decide that EMDR therapy might be a helpful approach, the client will embark on a journey through the eight phases of this therapy with their therapist by their side. During these sessions, the client will gently explore a negative image, belief, emotion, and physical sensation associated with a traumatic event. Together, the clinician and client will also work toward identifying a positive belief that signifies healing and resolution.

Typically, an EMDR therapy session lasts between 60 to 90 minutes, allowing for a safe and supportive environment to delve into these experiences. EMDR can be integrated with traditional talk therapy, offered as a complementary treatment with another therapist, or utilized as an independent approach to healing. The goal is always to support the client in their path to recovery and personal growth (EMDR International Association, 2022).

For clients that are in active eating disorders, we might need to pause trauma work if the eating disorder symptoms increase. The focus on the safe, calm place, and safety and containment skills becomes paramount. Those skills can also translate to helping eating disorder symptoms as well.

Acceptance and Commitment Therapy

Acceptance and commitment therapy (ACT) is a compassionate, evidence-based approach designed to support individuals grappling with eating disorders and trauma. Building on the principles of cognitive behavioral therapy, ACT recognizes that trying to control or suppress painful emotions can often make things feel even more difficult and distressing. Instead of solely focusing on changing an individual's thoughts, ACT invites them to engage in mindful behaviors, offering a gentle and effective alternative. This therapy can help with a range of challenges, including addiction, eating disorders, PTSD, depression, and obsessive compulsive disorder. Through its six core processes, ACT fosters psychological well-being and encourages individuals to embrace their experiences with kindness and understanding (Psychology Today, 2017). The six processes are:

1 Acceptance of emotions
2 Cognitive diffusion, which involves an individual changing the way they react but taking a step back to look at their reactions objectively

3 Being present
4 Self as context—an individual is more than their thoughts and feelings
5 Values—an individual identifies their values and strives to live by them
6 Committed Action—an individual takes concrete steps to put these things into action

Attachment Therapy

In Chapter 8, I reviewed Erikson's stages of development and the impact of chronic illness in "passing or failing" each phase of development. The attachment ruptures that may occur at one or more of these stages often need to be addressed directly in *attachment therapy*. People with attachment issues may have challenges in relationships. Attachment theory highlights how our early relationships with caregivers can shape the way we connect with others throughout our lives. When we face tough experiences in these early bonds, it can make it harder to build strong connections later in life.

The goal of attachment therapy is to guide people toward forming secure attachments. This can mean learning to trust your romantic partners and friends, managing any relationship anxiety that comes up, and working through past traumas in a supportive way. In attachment treatment, we examine childhood experiences that have caused trauma and work to understand how these traumas have led to issues in adult relationships. We aim to develop skills for emotional regulation in relationships and foster safe and meaningful connections with others (Effa, 2024).

Many individuals with a lifetime of chronic medical conditions struggle with attachment. With chronic illness, an individual may have repeated attachment ruptures in their adult relationships whether they are with family, friends, or a romantic partner. These compounded ruptures can lead to continued struggle in adult relationships as well as PTSD. Attachment therapy aims to repair attachment ruptures to lead to secure adult relationships.

Exploring Interoceptive Awareness

Interoceptive awareness is awareness of the body's sensations. When an individual is in a body with chronic illness or chronic pain, the sensation of pain can be scary. To cope and adapt, some may learn to ignore sensations of pain while others become hyperaware of discomfort and pain. A recent study sought to understand how interoception—the awareness of our internal bodily signals—might be impacted for those experiencing pain. The findings, which are significant, reveal that individuals living with chronic pain often face challenges with interoceptive accuracy while being more attuned to their internal sensations. This suggests that while they may be deeply aware of their bodily signals, they might struggle to interpret those signals accurately. This important insight highlights the complexity of living with chronic pain and emphasizes the need for more research in this area. It is crucial that we continue to explore these experiences to better support those affected (Horsburgh et al., 2024).

I can attest to this from my own experience, past and present. As I write this, I am experiencing pain in an area that was injured by a medical provider. When this pain started last week, I was full of fear and anxiety. I still have some fear attached to it. However, having the awareness of my body's cues also gives me access to the tools I need to address it. While it is uncomfortable physically and emotionally, if I have awareness of my body's sensations, I can tend to them. Just recently, my physical therapist and I discussed interoceptive awareness and cues as he taped my back.

Just as someone with an eating disorder is out of touch with their hunger and fullness cues, someone with chronic pain is often out of touch with pain and other physical sensations. It is important to have conversations with your treatment team to continue to assess and process these feelings and sensations. Although it can be scary to directly address pain, our pain is a signal that something may need to be tended to.

Progressive Desensitization to Recover from Body Image Disturbance

Progressive desensitization is not something that a clinician would traditionally use to work on body image, but it is helpful for body image disturbance with chronic illness because it is based on an actual "deformed" part of the body or scarring. This can help clients accept real changes in the body, not perceived or distorted changes. Someone may have new scarring, have lost a limb, and had other changes in their body as a result of a surgery, injury, or medical condition.

Progressive desensitization is a part of treatment for a phobia known as systematic desensitization in which the goal is to replace fear with relaxation. While we are not necessarily treating a true phobia, we need to work slowly to work through the anxiety. In systematic desensitization there are three steps, and the average length of treatment varies based on the number of fears as well as the intensity of each fear (Nash, 2022).

1 **Relaxation:** Clients are taught breathing and muscle relaxation techniques. Visualization of calming imagery or a safe calm place is often helpful.
2 **Creation of a fear hierarchy:** Clients create a list of their fears and rank them in order of lowest to highest level of anxiety and fear.
3 **Exposure:** This may start with visualizing the fear and working through the anxiety and response to it. We then move on to the fear itself and gradually expose clients to it while practicing relaxation techniques (Nash, 2022).

For example, my abdominal scar from surgery did not heal well; it was painful, developed keloids, and needed many treatments for the internal and external scarring, as well as the appearance. Today I do not love how it looks but I can accept it and look at it in the mirror. For quite some time after my surgery, it was distressing to look at. I would not look at it after a shower, and I would quickly get dressed so I did not have to see it. I needed to slowly expose myself to it as it was now a permanent part of me. I started with looking at it for 10 seconds, then 20, and so on. Sometimes I would cry, sometimes I would hold my breath. Over time, I was able to look at that scar with compassion, and I was no longer overly emotional at its appearance.

Accepting My Scars

December 14, 2018—1.5 months post-op and these are my 3 new scars; still healing.

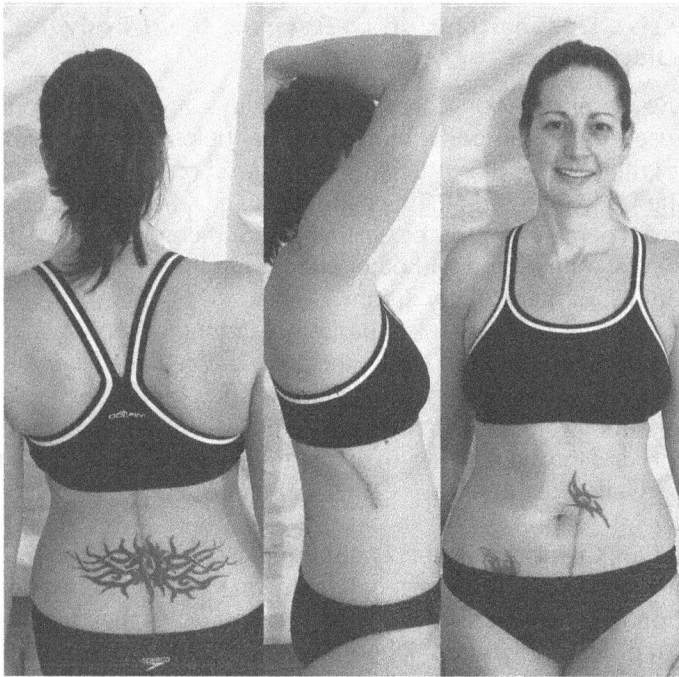

Accepting My Scars

Wearing My Scars Proudly

May 3, 2024—I wore this dress to show off my spine scar for the first time at the SOSORT (International Society on Scoliosis Orthopaedic Rehabilitation Treatment) International Congress.

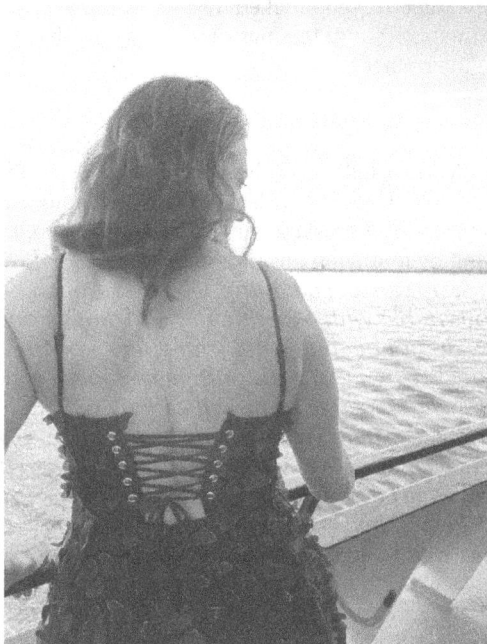

Wearing My Scars Proudly

Exercises for Clinicians

The following exercises utilize some of the treatment modalities described in this chapter for you to try with clients.

Exercise 10.1: Create a Containment Box

Individuals need a safe container to put their scary feelings and memories. In my early recovery, I created a safety and containment box, a tool that I have used with clients as well. This is where an individual makes a literal box to store feelings and memories to help them compartmentalize and process them as they move forward with treatment.

Guide clients to create their own containment box. They can find different boxes at a craft store; it can be a cigar box, or they might want a large box with a lock to keep those things contained under lock and key. This is very personal, and they have to do what feels right to them.

I have created several of my own containment boxes over the years. My very first one, which I still have, has a personalized collage on the outside and inside. On the top are images that are positive and hopeful, and inside are things that I wanted to "put away." Over time, I would write notes on slips of paper and also find images to put in the box. I put photos and other memories that I wanted to keep locked away. It was a safe way to acknowledge that these memories and feelings exist, and take their power away by keeping them in their place.

Exercise 10.2: Prompt for Narrative Therapy

What does an individual tell themselves about their body, their illness, and the place it holds in their life? In order for them to reauthor their lives, they need to know what their story is and what it means to them. Encourage them to do some writing by following this prompt.

Writing your story can feel daunting. Go into as much or as little detail as you feel comfortable with. As with all journaling and writing, please take breaks. You do not need to write your entire story in a day, week, or month. If you begin to feel anxious or triggered, please close your journal or your laptop and practice some self-care.

You need to honor where you are and pay attention to your emotions and distress. One technique is to write for 20 minutes, then take a break for 10 minutes. If you write for 20 minutes, you can come back to it in 10 minutes or in a few days. Remember, this is your recovery and there is no rush here. Rushing the process will serve to bring you more intense emotions and activation. What can you do to practice self-compassion here?

Once you do have your story written, you need to decide if you feel comfortable sharing it with someone and, if so, whom. This is where your support team and loved ones come in. You may not feel comfortable reading it out loud; however, it might feel safe to show it to someone and have them read it. This is vulnerable and scary, and you want to make sure you feel safe with the person who witnesses your story.

You can break it down and reassess it. Eating disordered or not, you rarely see yourself the way others see you, so an objective point of view can help here.

As with anything, starting neutral is the best approach. There is not an expectation to start with hating or disliking your body, illness, and struggles, and jump straight to saying that you love everything about yourself. That is not realistic. Cognitive behavior therapy tools may help you start to shift your thinking, which your clinician can talk to you about as you work through your narrative.

The goal for your narrative is to reduce your anxiety, fear, and sadness, and have a more neutral thought. So, instead of the thought being "I cannot stand to be in this body," you might be able to shift it to something more neutral, such as "Even though I am frustrated with my body at times, I can show my body compassion." An "even though" statement acknowledges both sides of your feelings. You need to validate your current feelings and allow room for other more neutral or positive thoughts.

I encourage you, on your own or with your therapist, to continue to explore using automatic thought records to find new statements that can release you from that negativity and create space for neutral statements and thoughts about your body. You do not have to hate the body that you were given. You also do not have to love it—neutrality is a wonderful goal.

Summary

There are various treatment modalities we use for addressing trauma and eating disorders. Before engaging in trauma work, it is essential to establish safety and containment with our clients. Some treatment modalities include narrative therapy, play therapy, EMDR, ACT, and progressive desensitization, which helps address body image disturbances resulting from illness, injury, or surgery. Play therapy is an effective approach for children diagnosed with medical trauma as well as PTSD. I shared some of my lived experiences to underscore the importance of these approaches. In the next chapter, I will discuss how to find a treatment team.

References

Effa, C. (2024, October 24). What to know about attachment-based therapy. Medical News Today. www.medicalnewstoday.com/articles/attachment-therapy#what-to-expect

EMDR International Association. (2022). About EMDR Therapy. www.emdria.org/about-emdr-therapy/

Horsburgh, A., Summers, S. J., Lewis, A., Keegan, R. J., & Flood, A. (2024). The relationship between pain and interoception: A systematic review and meta-analysis. *The Journal of Pain, 25*(7), 104476. https://doi.org/10.1016/j.jpain.2024.01.341

Locatelli, M. G. (2019). Play therapy treatment of pediatric medical trauma: A retrospective case study of a preschool child. *International Journal of Play Therapy, 29*(1), 33–42. https://doi.org/10.1037/pla0000109

Nash, J. (2022, September 23). Systematic Desensitization Steps: 13 Techniques & Worksheets. PositivePsychology.com. https://positivepsychology.com/systematic-desensitization/

Pietrangelo, A. (2019, October 11). Play therapy: What is it, how it works, and techniques. Healthline. www.healthline.com/health/play-therapy#when-its-used

Psychology Today. (2017). Acceptance and commitment therapy. www.psychologytoday.com/us/therapy-types/acceptance-and-commitment-therapy?msockid=08d5fa9535b867ba1ffeeb7134f766b8

Therapist.com. (2021, August 5). Play therapy: Definition, benefits, types, techniques. https://therapist.com/types-of-therapy/play-therapy

Vinney, C. (2019). What is narrative therapy? Definition and techniques. ThoughtCo. https://www.thoughtco.com/narrative-therapy-4769048

Chapter 11

From Specialists to Support: Key Steps in Finding the Ideal Medical Team

Eating disorder specialists typically agree that it is difficult to find medical providers who are educated and proficient in working with clients with eating disorders. At the primary care level, this is of paramount importance in recovery. Those with chronic medical conditions have many different medical providers, including specialists. For example, I have a spine surgeon, sports medicine doctor, physical therapist, and primary care physician. This year, I also worked with a hand surgeon when I had my race injury and needed surgery.

Therapeutic Alliance

The *therapeutic alliance* is a fundamental partnership between patients and medical providers where both take equal responsibility for medical care, progress, and outcomes. An alliance is defined as "a union or association formed for mutual benefit" (Oxford Advanced Learner's Dictonary, n.d.) It's interesting to see the words *mutual benefit* when it comes to a doctor/patient relationship. To me, it's a relationship just like any other we hope to have that includes trust, respect, communication, kindness, empathy, shared goals, and values (I have included a first-person narrative on the similarities between dating and finding a physical therapist later in this chapter, as it emphasizes the feelings and evolution of building a solid relationship).

Relationship-Focused Care

The medical profession is beginning to recognize that the doctor–patient relationship is essential for effective care. Instead of solely focusing on patient-centered approaches, clinicians are now prioritizing relationship-focused care. "Synergy is the physician-patient working alliance" (Fuertes et al., 2017).

Patient-centered care allows the patient to have a personal choice in their healthcare decisions based on their values, needs, and beliefs. The focus is on empathy and understanding rather than health directives (Grover et al.,

DOI: 10.4324/9781003500254-15

2022). Relationship-focused care is *also* patient-centered while allowing both the doctor and patient to be in the relationship.

In a recent conference presentation, Dr. Ovidio Bermudez discussed the importance of setting healthy expectations for both patient and physician. The physician needs to show up as a person in the relationship and allow the patient to get a sense of who they are. "How we show up matters" (Bermudez, 2024). In my personal experience, the humanness of my medical providers fosters trust and connection.

One study reviewed what led to patient adherence for treatment recommendations, and what researchers found is that compliance is attributed to a doctor's clear delivery and that patient's trust in them. There is also a connection with the patient's and doctor's secure attachment styles (Bennett et al., 2011). Physicians need to be reliable and consistent to establish a secure attachment with their patient.

Working with patients who have chronic medical conditions enables doctors and healthcare providers to develop special bonds with them. This relationship resembles a long-term partnership, which is different from the usual doctor–patient dynamic. Over time, this partnership becomes strong and meaningful. I often like to joke with my new physical therapists that we are in for a long-term relationship!

At the heart of this relationship is trust. Patients need to feel confident in their providers, follow their medical advice, and believe in their recommendations. They are also empowered to use their voice when a recommendation does not feel right. When this trust is established, it can lead to wonderful benefits for the patient, resulting in better long-term health outcomes and a greater quality of life.

It's also essential to recognize that patients are the true leaders in their own healthcare and recovery journeys. To build that trust, it's crucial for patients to feel seen, heard, and understood. Many of us have been patients for a long time, and we really know our bodies—every limitation, every ache, and every strength. If a patient doesn't feel as if they have a partnership with their provider, they might struggle to feel empowered and engaged in their treatment.

Collaboration with All Members of the Treatment Team

As eating disorder providers, it is normal practice to work as part of a multidisciplinary team, whether that is in a residential treatment setting or as an outpatient provider. That team will include a therapist, dietitian, and primary care physician, and may also include an eating disorder recovery coach, psychiatrist, and group therapist. Your client with a chronic illness likely has a number of specialists that they work with on a regular basis. For a client with an eating disorder and chronic illness, their team is expansive to include the specialist medical team as well any other adjunct supports, such as a personal trainer or a coach.

Feeling Gratitude for Strength and the Support of Others

November 28, 2019—I don't even know where to start with expressing my gratitude for this past year. This past year I recovered from my spine surgeries, I reconnected with so many friends, and I'm making great changes in my life! I'm excited to spend this holiday with my family!

I'm incredibly grateful for this woman here, Megan Cullen DPT, who helped me get strong before surgery and then taught me to walk and then run again. Today was my second Post Op 5K and I shaved a few seconds off of my time with my walk/run intervals. 37:51! Ankles are sore because they need to get stronger but other than that I have no pain in my back at all! I repeat, no pain in my back!

I am also grateful for Susan at GnR fitness which stands for grit and resilience! She pushes me and helps me get stronger every week! Had to represent today!

I'm grateful for all of you and your support! Have a wonderful Thanksgiving!

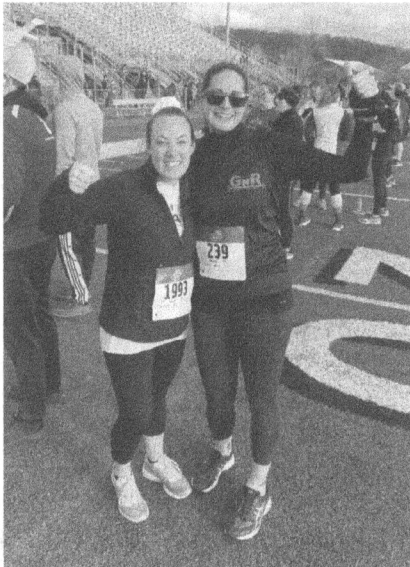

Tamie and Physical Therapist Megan Cullen PT, DPT

The Role of Physical Therapists in the Treatment of Chronic Illness

One person who may be on your client's medical team is a physical therapist. The role of physical therapists in the treatment of chronic illness is very therapeutic emotionally and physically. In some situations, finding a mental health provider is not an easy task, so other members of the medical team may fill that role, such as a physical therapist. Oftentimes, the physical therapist not only supports physical rehabilitation, but is also a sounding board for the many emotional challenges that often accompany illness, injury, surgery, and limb loss.

This emotional support becomes exponentially more important for those who have a chronic medical condition, and in some cases clients who have become adaptive athletes like me. I have complications from my spine and also from sports injuries. One of my physical therapists once told me that I'm "not the average bear," which made me feel validated, seen, heard and accepted.

How Is Physical Therapy Like Dating?

The following is a first-person narrative from my social media account @authortamiegangloff that explains how physical therapy can be like dating. A client may have concerns about their first meeting with a physical therapist, and the ongoing relationship needs to be built on trust and safety. As a clinician, consider how my experience may help direct clients to build their medical team.

Part 1: April 11, 2024

My good friend Stephanie has said that finding the right physical therapist is like finding a soul mate. And she's not wrong, I've had some amazing physical therapists in my life that have helped me so much, and they were really important relationships. And I moved on from them either because I moved out of the area or needed a different area of specialty.

I was telling a friend yesterday that I was meeting with a new physical therapist and I felt like I was going on a blind date because all of the same anxieties came up. Will they like me? Will they see my history and say, "Yikes, I don't want to go there"? Will this work? Will I be seen and understood?

So, I had my first appointment with this physical therapist, and we talked about our plan of action. And, also like dating, it was kind of painful. And it is going to be a lot of work.

I am looking forward to my second visit next week. I have been in physical therapy for over half of my life, and I know that it has always helped me. I am hopeful that I will get stronger and better and return to running and hiking and taking longer walks.

Part 2: May 30, 2024

I feel like I have developed a trusting relationship with my physical therapist, which is just as important for my mental health as it is for my physical health. I had a significant pain flare over the past couple of days and was feeling like I wanted to give up—I shared this with a friend to avoid falling into the trap of my anxiety and panic.

A physical therapist is someone that you see a couple of times per week. You are trusting them, and they are trusting that you are doing what you need to do at home, and you are being honest about your physical activities.

All of the physical therapists and physical therapist assistants are supportive, and I feel really held there. So, I feel like this relationship is working and I want to continue.

If you're nervous about your physical therapist relationship, talk to them about it. If we don't have that trusting relationship, we don't have anything.

I have been with this physical therapist for about two months now and we have made some progress and have had a little setback.

And it was frustrating for my body.

In relationships, we need to be open about our feelings and talk about potential solutions with each other. Physical therapists are an important relationship if you have a chronic medical condition, especially one that is musculoskeletal.

The relationship with your physical therapist is so important, and it is just something that is going to be a part of my life for a long time.

I went into physical therapy this morning, and when my physical therapist asked me how I was feeling, I said that I was frustrated with my body, and I described the pain that I was having and that it was more than it had been. He validated my feelings right away and assured me that we would continue to work on the solution and consider alternatives such as custom orthotics. He also showed a cool ice technique that worked! YAY! Another tool in my PT toolbox.

Remember, we have a team of people to help: friends, coaches, therapists (mental health and physical therapists), doctors, and so forth. We cannot recover from injury and surgery alone, and that includes the mental aspect. My friend asked me what a physiotherapist (physical therapist) can do to increase resilience. Patients see their physical therapists two to three times per week, far more than they see a psychotherapist or their physicians. A physical therapist can be a safe space, and they can listen and support you. A physical therapist should listen to your goals and make them their goals. You can then work on them together.

How Meaningful It Is to Have Your Medical Team Support You

December 15, 2023—So I just had the most amazing conversation with my sports medicine doctor, Dr. Payne. She shifted our conversation to what my future in sport will look like and then I got to determine what that is and advocate for myself and she encouraged me to try things I haven't done in a long time or to focus on something new, such as rock climbing, which sounds really exciting and fun. She also encouraged me to look at myself through the lens of a para-athlete and continue to modify and really make it my own. And that my future in sport doesn't have to look the same as anyone else's and that I can focus on joy and community. This is also a lot of what we talk about in eating disorder recovery so I really love that this is her perspective and this is such a meaningful conversation. I got an extra medal for her at my half marathon because I could not be where I am today without her and I'm so grateful. And if you do not have doctors in your life that make you feel this way, you should find other providers because we all need doctors that believe in us and support our goals.

Today marks five months since my accident and injury at Spartan Palmerton. I met Dr. Payne last summer when my spine was injured by a chiropractor, and having her in my life and in my corner has certainly changed my life so much for the better.

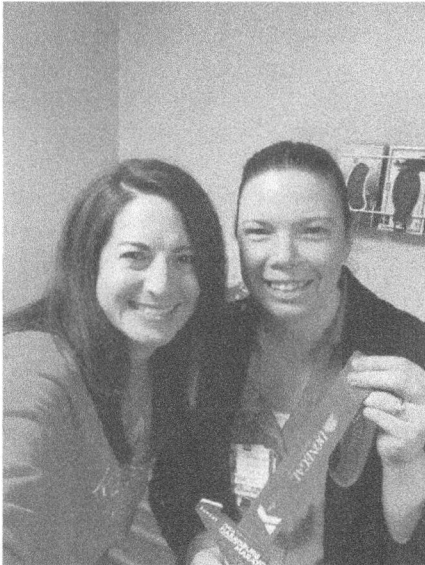

Tamie and Sports Medicine Doctor, Dr. Jennifer Payne

Bridging the Gap Between Disciplines

A critical aspect of treating chronic illness and eating disorders is in interdisciplinary training and understanding. As a field, we know that we need to continue to train across disciplines. There are a small number of physical therapists and strength and conditioning coaches as well as personal trainers who are specialized in working with eating disorders. A small percentage of spine doctors and sports medicine doctors have training and experience working with eating disorders. Postgraduate education is necessary in all fields, but there is not mandated training for every medical discipline regarding eating disorders during that time.

Although it is important for us to empower our patients to communicate with their medical treatment teams, it is equally important for us as eating disorder specialists, to be there to help educate those providers. That collaboration is so important. For example, if you have a client with an eating disorder who's going in for a spine surgery or seeing a sports medicine doctor for a tendon injury from playing soccer, they can reach out and be that first touch point to explain more about their client's eating disorder and how the medical team can support them together. From my experience as an eating disorder specialist, I don't expect the sports medicine doctor to be trained in meal planning for an eating disorder because that's the role of the dietitian. The dietitian doesn't have to know how the spine is reconstructed—that's for the spine surgeon to know. It is the eating disorder clinician's responsibility to reach out to those specialists in different lanes to help a client create a comprehensive treatment experience.

Here's one way those in other lanes of the treatment team can learn about eating disorders. In 2024, I presented at a scoliosis conference. I am not a medical provider, so it was important to me to bring eating disorders and body image education to spine professionals. As clinicians, we need to continue to train and educate those in other disciplines so we can provide the best care for our clients. There is progress being made in training medical professionals specifically for eating disorders within the school setting. For example, I teach an eating disorder psychology class to students. However, most of us had very little eating disorder education in our formal university education, and that is true for doctors, physical therapists, dietitians, and coaches.

As both a clinician and educator, I will stand on my soapbox and talk to anyone who will listen, whether it is educating the scoliosis world about eating disorders and body image or if it is educating the spine doctor's office as to why they do not need to weigh me before a spine injection. It can be scary, even as a clinician, to use my voice. I try to remember that I have to continue to use my voice, always, for the person who has not yet found their voice.

Scope of Practice

Scope of practice varies across disciplines as well as state of licensure and it continues to evolve and change. This is important to consider for multi-disciplinary treatment of chronic illness and eating disorders.

Physicians have the most strict scope of practice guidelines. The Federation of State Medical Boards defines scope of practice as:

> the rules, the regulations, and the boundaries within which a fully qualified practitioner with substantial and appropriate training, knowledge, and experience may practice in a field of medicine or surgery, or other specifically defined field. Such practice is also governed by requirements for continuing education and professional accountability.
>
> (Newlon et al., 2022)

It is important for me to stress practice guidelines because, as I shared in Chapter 8, I was injured by a medical provider. Although she claimed to be able to treat me, it is likely that it was not within her scope of practice to treat complicated spine conditions.

Regulation of medical providers is complex, and I believe it should be more specific. For example, a chiropractor may receive insurance payment for manipulating the spine; however, there is no specific scope of practice regarding specific conditions such as scoliosis or a postoperative fused spine (Commonwealth of Pennsylvania, 2024). More specific scope of practice could prevent injury and harm done to patients.

The hope is that providers do not practice outside of their scope. Eating disorders are a very specific and nuanced specialty. Those of us who treat eating disorders have specialized training with continuing education focusing on this specialty. There are certifications that focus on eating disorder treatment and more specific certifications based on diagnosis. A clinician treating eating disorders, without training, is working outside their scope of practice, and that is unethical. It is important for a clinician to fully assess clients to determine if they are within your scope of practice and if you are the best fit for the client. If you are not the best fit, you should refer the client to the proper specialist (DeAngelis, 2018).

Suggestions for Clinicians

Clients need to be empowered to ask to have their needs met by their medical team. As we know, many of our clients have experienced medical traumatic stress and negative experiences in a medical setting. Asking to have their needs met might be scary and intimidating. As we discussed in Chapter 8, many of our clients are experiencing PTSD from their medical experiences and continue to be hypervigilant, often looking for fault or leaving appointments not being seen and heard, left feeling hurt and angry.

We need to continue to assess where our clients are in their trauma work and prepare for medical appointments accordingly. The following exercises can help you work with a client who is getting ready to see a provider.

Exercise 11.1: Questions to Ask Clients Preparing for a Medical Appointment

Clients should let you know when they have upcoming appointments so you can help them prepare. We can ask questions including:

1 Is this a new provider?
2 How do you feel about this doctor going into this appointment?
3 What are your current feelings about your illness and/or pain?
4 What questions do you need to have answered?
5 Let's work on creating a list together to bring in to your appointment.
6 Do you feel equipped to ask your questions?
7 Can we practice role-playing your questions?
8 Do you feel like you need to bring someone into your appointment with you?
9 Can you record your appointment so you can listen afterward when you are not feeling as activated?

Exercise 11.2: Prepare Your Client to Interview New Medical Providers

Clients should interview potential doctors, physical therapists, coaches, and other medical providers to make sure they are the best fit and ensure that their training, skillset, and scope of practice meet the needs of the client. Not all professionals are bound by ethical standards of scope of practice. Help your client make sure their condition is within the provider's capacity and expertise, and that the provider can meet their needs. You can have them:

1 Ask for referrals for friends/family/colleagues.
2 Create a list of questions to ask potential providers/specialists:

   • What is your specific training in X diagnosis?
   • Do you belong to any professional organizations dedicated to training and education of X diagnosis?
   • How many years of experience do you have with this patient population?
   • How often do you perform this procedure/surgery?

3 Research experience and patient outcomes. There are several websites dedicated to reviews of doctors; have your clients read patient reviews. These include:

   • Vitals
   • Healthgrades
   • Birdeye
   • WebMD
   • Rater8
   • Healthline

4 Get a second opinion and a third or fourth one.
5 Comfort and fit is equally as important as experience. Your client should consider what they are looking for in a provider by considering the following:

- Do you have a preference for your physician's gender?
- Do you have an age preference?
- What personality are you most comfortable with?

Summary

Research and experience teach us that a therapeutic alliance and relationship-focused care are best for the patient and treatment outcomes. I shared social media posts about how physical therapy is like dating to highlight the strong relational aspects of working with a physical therapist. As clinicians, we can serve as advocates for our clients and work collaboratively with their medical teams. We can bridge the educational gap between disciplines by educating providers on eating disorders and our clients' eating disorder struggles. We can prepare our clients to find medical providers to meet their needs and serve as a guide in this journey.

References

Bennett, J. K., Fuertes, J. N., Keitel, M., & Phillips, R. (2011). The role of patient attachment and working alliance on patient adherence, satisfaction, and health-related quality of life in lupus treatment. *Patient Education and Counseling, 85*(1), 53–59. https://doi.org/10.1016/j.pec.2010.08.005

Bermudez, O. (2024, October 25). Adventures in Treating Eating Disorders: Sharing Wisdom from a Cumulative 75 Years of Practice. [Conference presentation]. Renewed Conference, Franking TN, United States.

Commonwealth of Pennsylvania. (2024). 55 Pa. Code Chapter 1145. Chiropractors' Services. www.pacodeandbulletin.gov/Display/pacode?file=/secure/pacode/data/055/chapter1145/chap1145toc.html

DeAngelis, T. (2018, May). What should you do if a case is outside your skill set? American Psychological Association. www.apa.org/monitor/2018/05/ce-corner

Fuertes, J. N., Toporovsky, A., Reyes, M., & Osborne, J. B. (2017). The physician-patient working alliance: Theory, research, and future possibilities. *Patient Education and Counseling, 100*(4), 610–615. https://doi.org/10.1016/j.pec.2016.10.018

Grover, S., Fitzpatrick, A., Azim, F. T., Ariza-Vega, P., Bellwood, P., Burns, J., Burton, E., Fleig, L., Clemson, L., Hoppmann, C. A., Madden, K. M., Price, M., Langford, D., & Ashe, M. C. (2022). Defining and implementing patient-centered care: An umbrella review. *Patient Education and Counseling, 105*(7), 1679–1688. https://doi.org/10.1016/j.pec.2021.11.004

Newlon, J. L., Murphy, E. M., Ahmed, R., & Illingworth, K. S. (2022). Determining and regulating scope of practice for health care professionals: A participatory, multiple stakeholder approach. *Research in Social and Administrative Pharmacy, 19*(3). https://doi.org/10.1016/j.sapharm.2022.11.005

Oxford Advanced Learner's Dictionary. (n.d.) Alliance. www.oxfordlearnersdictionaries.com/definition/english/alliance

Chapter 12

Sports Injury Versus Chronic Medical Condition—What's the Difference?

In 2023, I injured myself significantly while participating in an obstacle course race. This resulted in months of rehabilitation. During my recovery from this sports-related injury and surgery, I realized that I essentially felt the same emotions with a severe sports injury as I did throughout my spine surgeries. I realized that I could use sports injury psychology as a modality to help those with chronic medical conditions.

There are some great books and treatment modalities available on sports psychology and, even more specifically, sports injury psychology. The more I read during my own recovery, the more I found parallels between sports injury and chronic medical conditions. This disappointing and frustrating event in my personal life turned into a teachable moment that brought darkness into the light, just like many of my other health obstacles over the years.

Clinicians should consider looking into sports psychology to treat their clients living with chronic illnesses and even those with eating disorders. Even if a client is not particularly active, the obstacles they face with their chronic illness may feel much like recovery from a sports injury. In this chapter, I will highlight some of the more useful sports psychology strategies I have found as well as share my personal story and the story of Hope as it relates to the topic.

What Can We Learn from Sports Injury Psychology?

Importance of Social Support

Many studies have shown that injured athletes who receive strong *social support* from influential figures, such as coaches, tend to have a more satisfying rehabilitation experience and experience lower levels of anxiety and depression. Conversely, a lack of support from teammates and coaches can create additional challenges during recovery. This highlights the importance of carefully examining the different sources and aspects of social support, as they play a vital role in helping athletes heal both emotionally and physically (Tranaeus et al., 2024). Social support is crucial to quality of life in those who are adaptive

DOI: 10.4324/9781003500254-16

athletes as well as athletes who do not have disabilities. Social support can be found in the forms of emotional support, encouragement, guidance, and tangible support, such as helping with tasks (Mira et al., 2023).

In eating disorder and substance use recovery, we talk a lot about community, whether that's a support group or a 12-step meeting. For athletes, loss of sport can mean loss of community and loss of identity, so it is important to maintain that social support even in the midst of injury and illness. We know that so much can happen in the group dynamic, which is why it's such a big part of our eating disorder treatment programs at all levels of care. This is a place where clients can relate to their peers and feel supported by them as well as by the clinicians leading a group. Consider your client's needs and whether or not they may be feeling estranged from their social support as they grapple with injury or other symptoms of their chronic illness and eating disorder. Finding the right connections could really improve their treatment plan.

Physical and Emotional Readiness to Return to Sport May Not Occur at the Same Time

It is important to acknowledge that physical and emotional readiness might not occur at the same time. There is often a fear of reinjury or not being able to return to pre-injury abilities. The coach, physical therapist, physician, and mental health provider can work together to ensure a client is ready to return to sport.

I see a strong connection here between the athlete returning to sport and the patient returning to activity after a surgery, flare, or setback. The fear of a negative outcome may prevent someone from going to physical therapy, adhering to treatment recommendations, and returning to their lives. Athlete or not, this is applicable to your client.

Developing Fear as a Result of Injury

If someone has experienced a traumatic sports injury or has a disability as the result of a traumatic incident such as a car accident, they may develop fears that are potentially life-limiting. For example, if an individual develops a fear of driving or even being in a car after an accident, that can lead to a refusal to drive or be driven. That can place a lot of limits on their life and independence. Similarly, an athlete may have a fear of returning to their sport or exercise in general after injury. The fear of accidents is known as *dystychiphobia*; treatment modalities include those that we have already covered including CBT, mindfulness, and systematic desensitization (Cleveland Clinic, n.d.). As a personal example, I developed a fear of falling after my race accident in 2023.

Sports Injury-Related Growth

Injured athletes are more likely to experience growth and positive life changes if they can rally support and resources, whether tangible help with tasks or emotional and spiritual support. In one study, to help facilitate this growth, researchers recommended participants follow a *narrative approach*, including encouraging the athlete to share their story, understand the context of their story, ask directive questions to help change the narrative, take action on identified opportunities, and then name their growth and share it with others (Wadey et al., 2019). This type of approach is common in the many books and documentaries by athletes that report how they have overcome seemingly impossible odds.

When an athlete begins to notice positive changes—not only in their physical condition but also in their overall biopsychosocial well-being—it can be a truly uplifting experience. These improvements can touch every aspect of their life, extending far beyond the confines of their injury or sport. With the right support and a proactive mindset, this phase can be a remarkable opportunity for transformation and personal growth. It's important to recognize that *resilience* is a key part of this journey. It reflects an individual's ability to adapt to stress, pain, and the limitations they may face while finding acceptance for their current situation and emotions. Embracing resilience can empower an individual to focus on solutions and remain open to their experiences, which can be incredibly liberating. This growth can manifest as a new perspective, the development of healthier coping strategies, or even new positive life choices that align with their values and aspirations. An individual must remember that they are not alone in this journey, and each small step forward is significant (McKay, 2022). The clinician can remind a client of this and encourage them to see adversity not as a threat but as a challenge (McKay, 2022).

My Experience with Sports Injury

Prior to my spine surgeries, as I had more pain and limitations, I would listen to my well-meaning athlete friends as they would share their sports injuries and say that they could relate. "When I tore my Achilles …" "When I sprained my ankle …" I would get so frustrated and roll my eyes (not to their face, of course). Not that their experience wasn't valid, but it wasn't the same as mine, living with scoliosis my entire life. Sure, their pain was real, but it was only temporary. There was no way they could *get* me. I truly assumed that it must have been easier on them. Then I would see them return to sports and running and presume that it had been effortless. I get that it is always a challenge to recover and get back to it, but I couldn't imagine that they could relate to my condition.

I learned the hard way that they could *in fact* relate. In July 2023, after years spent regaining strength following my spine surgery, I endured my first serious race injury. I slipped off an obstacle during a Spartan race; the obstacle was beater, which are monkey bars that move. I was crushing it, and then, as I reached for the bell, my left hand slipped. I had a hard landing and broke my wrist in four places as well as my clavicle. I went to the ER at the local hospital and was told that I needed surgery. I texted photos of my x-rays to my trusted orthopedic friends, and they agreed that surgery was the only option. I had no time to stress about the surgery, as it was scheduled for the next day.

The surgery went well, and I returned home to recover. I live alone so there were some significant challenges. I needed a lot of help. My perception of that recovery was definitely skewed. My major spine surgeries took me about nine months to recover from—that is, from day of surgery to when I could return to running. This was only one surgery (with some more titanium), so I assumed the recovery would be much shorter. That's logical, right? Six weeks later, I learned that my clavicle was also fractured. I was still having pain in my shoulder, so I told my sports medicine doctor, and she ordered a STAT MRI and we discovered that I had a non-displaced clavicle fracture. I felt defeated and deflated. My recovery was longer and more painful than I could have imagined.

Celebrating the Small Wins

January 5, 2024—I am smiling, and I was crying, like I crossed the finish line. I was smiling so big as I carried this case of water up the stairs because I haven't done this in so long, and we are now just shy of 6 months after my race injury and surgery. I am still recovering and still in PT and will be for quite a while, but it felt so good to cross that finish line with a case of water tonight!

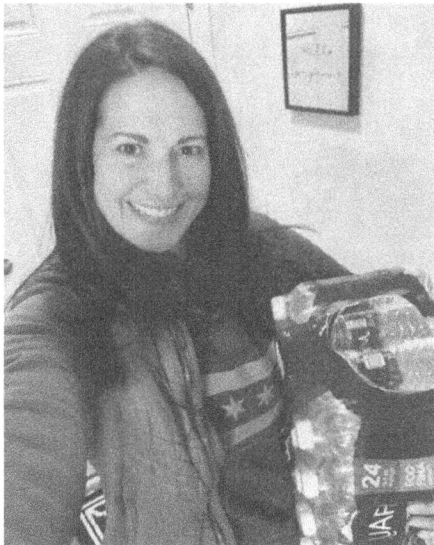

Celebrating the Small Wins

I began to struggle mentally with the inability to move my body the way I wanted to. I felt the frustration of not being able to drive, my employer being unhappy with me, the inability to sleep due to pain, feeling alone and isolated, and fear of the future. Altogether, I started to realize that the feelings I was having were not only similar to what I felt throughout my spine surgeries and recovery, but they were the same. The anxiety, mood swings, unknowns—they were all the same, and it was rough.

As mentioned earlier, I did develop a fear of falling and injury as a result of this race accident. I still have not fully overcome this fear, but I have begun to work on it by practicing climbing in a safe, indoor environment. This was at the recommendation of my sports medicine doctor.

Trying Something New

February 10, 2024—Well, friends! This is been a long recovery from Spartan Palmerton 7 months ago. My PT and sports med doc have suggested trying rock climbing, so I went to @spookynooksports today and was a little surprised at the level of anxiety I felt trying to go up that wall! I was patient with myself and took breaks and used some self-talk. I checked the self-belay about 5 times each time before I went up and I got some support of the lovely people that were in the gym and kept going until I got a blister on my finger! I am super proud of my effort, and working through my anxiety and getting stronger!

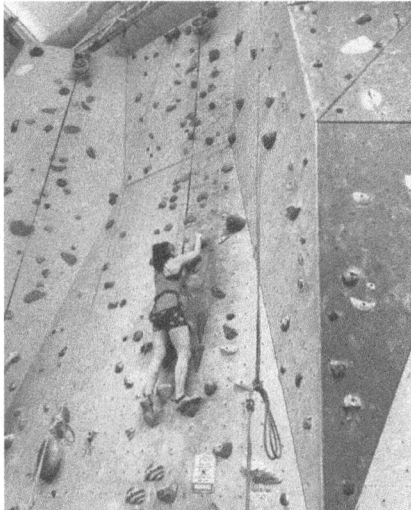

Trying Something New

At a recent conference, I was asked, as an athlete, how I was treated differently with my sports injury versus my chronic illness. This was tricky to answer. I was treated poorly by an employer when I had my major sports injury. It felt almost as if, since I "did it to myself," I didn't deserve sympathy. I did what I could to advocate for myself and then I ultimately left that employer for that reason specifically. I figured that if I was going to be treated poorly for a sports injury and surgery, I would not want to find out how I would be treated if I needed time off for a surgery related to my disability. My friends, family, and teammates were extremely supportive throughout my spine surgeries and my wrist surgery and lengthy recovery. The nature of my surgery wasn't relevant to my loved ones who supported me no matter what.

There are many athletes with disabilities, so I was intrigued by this question and contemplated it more broadly. Sports injury can be seen as a rite of passage. Athletes support one another, and the community is like no other. That is my personal experience in triathlon, open-water swimming, running, and obstacle course racing. When one of us is injured, we support each another. Injured athletes often show up at a race to cheer for their teammates who are not injured. There are social media groups dedicated to sports, and I have made some friends when I shared about my race injuries.

The longer you are an athlete, the more prone you are to injury. As Dr. Payne recently put it, if you are 49 and an athlete, you are going to get injured! For me, most of my limitations are related to my spine, surgeries, or my neck limitations. I have worked hard to adapt and overcome these limitations. *It is important for an individual to keep in mind that a sports injury can wreak just as much havoc on your life as a chronic medical condition.*

Athletes with Disabilities

A study by Mira et al. (2023), "Well-being, Resilience and Social Support of Athletes with Disabilities: A Systematic Review," examines the role of sport for people with disabilities. Sport plays a positive role in well-being, resilience, social support, confidence, and quality of life of those with disabilities. People with motor disabilities who practice sport have higher life satisfaction compared to people with motor disabilities who do not practice sport. A motor disability is a condition that hinders sensation or movement. Also of note in this study is the importance of social support.

Individuals with disabilities should continue to speak with their treatment team about their activities and what they would like to do. What an individual person can or cannot do is unique to their condition. For example, during a recent webinar, I was asked if some activities could increase a curve or illness. I could not provide a blanket answer to this question. Everyone's body is so different. Even within the same disease process or progression, what an individual is able to do differs. In my own life, I talk to my doctors and physical therapists about this. Part of staying ahead of injury and keeping the positive mental aspect of sport means that an individual is responsible for ensuring that they are not causing further complications because of their sports and movement. As a clinician, you may be able to help advise a client, but they should also talk to other members of their treatment team to make sure they are engaging in safe and appropriate levels of activity for their condition.

Profile: Hope—Wheelchair Athlete, ARFID, Advocate, Mental Health Coach, Paraplegic

Hope is a force; she is an inspiration. Oftentimes when we meet someone like her, we don't truly see all of the layers underneath and the grit and challenges she has gone through to get where she is. I followed her on social media first, and later I was able to meet her through a mutual friend. We initially Facetimed, and I became a complete fangirl! In preparation for my Spartan race, Hope reminded me that if she could race in a wheelchair, I could do it with metal in my spine. She says, "I'm a Spartan; I've got this."

Hope became paralyzed at the age of 21 as a result of domestic violence, and her life changed in an instant. As a result of that significant life alteration, she developed avoidant restrictive food intake disorder (ARFID) because of the changes to her daily life and gastrointestinal system. Hope developed a fear of what can happen when she eats. As she says, "Digestion is awful." She was diagnosed with gastroesophageal reflux disease (GERD) and takes medication to manage that. However, as a paraplegic, her sphincter does not close all the way. If she eats too much, she will vomit when she bends over, and this is involuntary. She states that this is painful and awful, and she will do whatever she can to not allow it to happen. Her eating disorder is a result of her disability. While she may get comments about her size, her eating concerns are unrelated to her appearance.

In our discussion about her eating disorder, Hope stated that she thought that this fear was a thing outside of spinal cord injuries. She had no idea that ARFID was an actual diagnosis. While the reasons for developing it may be different in individuals, ARFID has many causes and presentations. ARFID can cause someone to limit food intake out of fear of what might happen when they eat. Oftentimes, ARFID is caused by trauma, anxiety, and fear. This is true for Hope.

Hope knows many people in her spinal cord community who won't leave their home because they are afraid of what will happen when they eat. "I get terrified. When I have a gas pain, I am afraid. I might end up with diarrhea because of the anxiety around it." So much of her life is planned around having to go to the bathroom, where she can cath herself (this refers to the use of a straight catheter to help her urinate), or if she will be close to a bathroom if she needs to have a bowel movement.

Despite the challenges of ARFID, Hope continues to push herself and live life on her own terms. She climbed to the summit of Mount Kilimanjaro in 2022 to raise awareness for suicide in the disability community. During this climb, she was not able to nourish herself sufficiently out of fear of not being able to go to the bathroom while on the mountain. "I was starving myself because I was terrified." She was able to complete the climb, but she knew that it was dangerous. Breathing at that altitude takes a lot of energy, and she lacked appropriate energy because of her calorie deficit during the climb.

During this quest, Hope met the love of her life and has been married now for two years and lives a very busy, peaceful, and happy life in Tanzania.

She and her husband have worked together to handle her anxieties around eating, as food is a highly important part of Tanzanian culture. Her husband's family show their love and care for her with food, and she struggled at first with them as she could not eat the amount she was served. She really wanted to connect and enjoy the time with her new family, but her anxiety of eating overpowered the joy of the experience. With the support of her husband, she has started to overcome her fears surrounding food. Her husband will plate food for her if they are with family and order food for her when they are out. The food is very different there, farm to table and organic, and she feels that, after an initial month, her body feels much better, and she is able to feel more normal with her gastrointestinal concerns. The food, support, and peace in Tanzania have been very healing for her.

Hope is a mental health coach and works with clients with trauma, disabilities, and spinal cord injuries. She is a Spartan and runs three businesses. She is committed to helping others and is grateful that everything she does helps someone. Her obstacle course racing team races together, lifts (literally) each other up, and supports one another. As she says, "We are all a team; it's not just me in the wheelchair." Everyone on the team has a disability whether it is invisible, visible, cognitive, or emotional.

Activities for Clinicians

Goal Setting—SMART Goals

The SMART (specific, measurable, achievable, relevant, and time-bound) acronym is believed to have been introduced in November 1981 in Spokane, Washington. It was coined by George T. Doran, a consultant and former director of corporate planning for Washington Water Power Company. He shared his insights in a paper titled "There's a S.M.A.R.T. Way to Write Management's Goals and Objectives" (Haughey, 2014). Since then, many fields have adopted it for goal setting and self-improvement, including addiction medicine and behavioral health.

As clinicians, we help clients to ensure that these goals aren't too broad or unrealistic. Goal setting helps with emotion regulation because individuals adopt expectations that are set realistically. This approach is an *active coping skill*. Typically, those who use active coping skills during injury recovery have a better recovery outcome. This same modality works in recovery from extensive surgery, a flare, or a setback due to a chronic medical condition. We also utilize this in recovery from an eating disorder as well as co-occurring substance use and mental health disorders. See Exercise 12.1 at the end of this chapter for examples of how a client might use SMART goals.

How Does This Come Together for Clients with Chronic Illness and Eating Disorders?

I have found that all of this can apply to eating disorder recovery. Clients with eating disorders have fears and phobias; they can develop a fear of movement whether that is going back to a sport that might have been triggering and making the choice to no longer participate in a sport that is focused on weight. SMART goals are essential in recovery from illness and an eating disorder. Without small and achievable goals, this is too overwhelming.

Many clients aim to be the perfect client and want to do recovery perfectly. SMART goals help to break those goals down into small bites that are manageable. Highlighting the support recommended in sports injury psychology, clients may need emotional support or tangible support such as friends and family to eat meals with or support with tasks such as grocery shopping or meal prep. The importance of community and "team" resonates with our clients as well, which is why we utilize group therapy in higher levels of care, and it is recommended for ongoing support as well. A client with an eating disorder experiences anxiety of returning to "real life" after being in a higher level of care and away from work or school. We need to have a plan in place for how we can slowly integrate them back into work, school, and social engagements.

Exercise 12.1: SMART Goal Examples

The following can be used as a script to guide a client through setting SMART goals:

If you have not utilized SMART goals, let's take a closer look. You can do this with your therapist, physiotherapist, or on your own. First, let me tell you what SMART stands for: SMART = specific, measurable, achievable, realistic, and time-bound.

Let's look at a few examples of how this might work for eating disorders and chronic illness.

Example 1: You are currently completing 50 percent of your meal plan and would like to work up to 100 percent meal completion. This takes time and is a process. An example of SMART goals for this could be to take it one week at a time or one day at a time.

> *S—You will slowly increase meal plan intake by increasing to 60 percent of your meal plan this week.*
> *M—You will track your meal completion through your recovery app to share with your therapist and dietitian.*
> *A—You will progress slowly so this is an achievable goal.*
> *R—You will increase your plan by 10 percent a week, which is more realistic than getting to 100 percent in a week.*
> *T—You will only measure for a week and can reevaluate this goal for next week.*

Example 2: You are an injured runner who has completed physical therapy and would like to train for a half marathon.

> S—*You will create a specific training plan to slowly work up to a half marathon, which will happen slowly and incrementally with daily, weekly and monthly goals.*
> M—*You will track your progress with your coach or physical therapist on an app such as Training Peaks or Strava.*
> A—*Your goals will be small and incremental, likely beginning with run/walk intervals, slowly increasing your amount of run time and mileage; the expectation is to not return to full running and to work with a slow progression instead.*
> R—*You will not be ready for your half marathon in a month—realistic is a slow progression, following your plan and listening to your body.*
> T—*You will follow your 8–12-week plan to get ready for race day.*

You can utilize this approach for any injury, illness, or eating disorder. For example, after a surgery, this might mean that you are going to walk every day for ten minutes; for other people, this might mean they're going to sign up for a race in a few months to work toward that goal.

Summary

Sports injury psychology has many components that can be directly applied and translated to our work with clients who have eating disorders and chronic illnesses. The importance of community and social support is critical for all of these populations. Clients may develop a fear of returning to work, school, or sport. Sports injury-related growth is the same thing that happens when someone overcomes their eating disorder or recovers from a major surgery or setback. They now are able to see positive changes in their lives that extend far beyond recovery from illness. We can help foster this in our clients. We can support our clients by working with them to change their narrative and set SMART goals and continue to work to ensure that they are reasonable goals. In the next section of this book, I address strategies for individuals to use while living with chronic conditions and managing eating disorders.

References

Cleveland Clinic. (n.d.). Dystychiphobia (fear of accidents). https://my.clevelandclinic.org/health/diseases/22604-dystychiphobia-fear-of-accidents
Haughey, D. (2014, December 13). A brief history of SMART goals. Project Smart. www.projectsmart.co.uk/smart-goals/brief-history-of-smart-goals.php
Mckay, C. (2022). *The Mental Impact of Sports Injury*. CRC Press.

Mira, T., Costa, A. M., Jacinto, M., Diz, S., Monteiro, D., Rodrigues, F., Matos, R., & Antunes, R. (2023). Well-being, resilience and social support of athletes with disabilities: A systematic review. *Behavioral Sciences, 13*(5), 389. https://doi.org/10.3390/bs13050389

Tranaeus, U., Gledhill, A., Johnson, U., Podlog, L., Wadey, R., Diane Wiese Bjornstal, & Ivarsson, A. (2024). 50 years of research on the psychology of sport injury: A consensus statement. *Sports Medicine, 54*, 1733–1748. https://doi.org/10.1007/s40279-024-02045-w

Wadey, R., Roy-Davis, K., Evans, L., Howells, K., Salim, J., & Diss, C. (2019). Sport psychology consultants' perspectives on facilitating sport injury-related growth. *The Sport Psychologist, 33*(3), 244–255. https://doi.org/10.1123/tsp.2018-0110

Part 5

How Individuals Can Live with Chronic Illness and Manage Eating Disorders

The final section of this book, Part 5, focuses on living with chronic illness, specifically concerning how to manage energy reserves, health anxiety, and fear of the future. I will explore the concept of movement in various ways, including the benefits of movement, defining healthy movement, the experiences of adaptive athletes, and addressing the fear of movement.

I will also discuss the impact of chronic illness on relationships, drawing insights from Agamemnon and Zephyr's lived experience as a couple. Additionally, I will tackle other relational issues that can occur while dating and maintaining friendships. This section will conclude with a discussion on resilience—how it is defined and how it can be developed. I will cover topics such as values, joy, and quality of life.

Each chapter will include relevant research findings and end with practical suggestions for clinicians. I will add anecdotes from my personal story as it pertains to the topics discussed.

- Chapter 13: Managing Energy Reserves for Chronic Illness and Eating Disorders
- Chapter 14: The Spectrum of Movement: From Fear to Joy
- Chapter 15: Impact of Chronic Illness on Relationships
- Chapter 16: Resilience and Quality of Life

DOI: 10.4324/9781003500254-17

Managing Energy Reserves for Chronic Illness and Eating Disorders

Those who struggle with chronic medical conditions grapple with fear of the future and anxiety over when the other shoe will drop. They struggle with limited energy, often overextending themselves to overcompensate for perceived shortcomings. Let's take a closer look at how this impacts an individual.

In one study, researchers interviewed patients with Crohn's disease, focusing on the experiences of those living with chronic illness outside of the elderly population. Some participants were able to work outside the home, while others expressed a fear of the future. Notably, just 25 percent of the individuals were able to accept their diagnosis and move forward in their lives without fear and anxiety. Every participant talked about living with fatigue and limited energy, emphasizing the importance of approaching life one day at a time. These findings can also resonate with individuals dealing with other chronic illnesses (Natale & Pai, 2021).

Consider Spoon Theory

One helpful strategy for those living with chronic illnesses is to think of energy in terms of spoons. *Spoon theory* was developed by blogger Christine Miserandino, who lives with lupus, as a way of describing her experience to her partner. One day, she and her partner were sitting at a table, and she glanced at the spoons, and it occurred to her that she could use them to describe how she feels every day. She told her partner that each day she has a certain number of spoons to use, and every day is different based on many factors such as daily activities planned, current symptoms and pain, stress, sleep, recovery from a recent flare or treatment, and so much more (About Christine Miserandino, n.d.). This language to describe energy reserves has taken on a life of its own in the chronic illness community, and many people find spoon theory useful.

Everyone has different energy reserves to use each day based on their illness and life. An individual might work two jobs, be a new mother, or have a long day at work. An individual may have 20 spoons one day or feel like they have limitless spoons! The next day they might feel as if they only have the energy

DOI: 10.4324/9781003500254-18

to shower, fold their laundry, and run to Target for some coffee creamer, which would likely translate to a day with a small number of spoons.

This is a language that all "spoonies" share. I could tell a friend with a chronic illness that I have no spoons left for today and they would know exactly what that meant. My non-spoonie friends probably do not understand what that means; however, I do believe that everyone knows what having no spoons feels like. We have all had family emergencies, illness, loss in the family, struggles, and challenges that left us feeling depleted with nothing left to give. That is the everyday way of life for those with chronic illness.

Personally, some days I can run a half marathon, speak at a conference, enjoy a night out with friends, and clean my apartment. Those are days with lots of spoons. On other days, I might work from my bed with my laptop, not wash my hair, and only manage to clean the litter box and feed the cats. I would describe these low-energy days as having very few or no spoons. On the days that I am traveling and using more spoons, I usually pay the price later, meaning that I know that I will have an increase in pain or have less energy (fewer spoons) in the days that follow. If I use more spoons than I have, I may experience a pain flare that keeps me in bed with my ice packs or a heating pad in the middle of the night.

Searching for More Spoons

May 2024—I need more spoons! I am in the middle of an epic few weeks that includes presenting a poster at an international scoliosis conference, advocating at my nation's capitol regarding eating disorder legislation, and now heading to an eating disorder conference, followed by a body-positive fitness conference this weekend. That quote, "all of the women in me are tired" has new meaning today. I typically never travel back-to-back weeks, and this is the third week and my body is telling me. It is yelling, you have no spoons, you are negative so many spoons that we can't count that high!

Movement is medicine so my usual plan to work out in between trips has worked against me because, since I am traveling more, my body needs more recovery time. I am not recovering from my travel or my workouts. So much that I woke up with pain in my jaw from clenching my jaw. So, what can I do now? I started by letting my co-workers and co-presenters know. That way, if I need extra help, I can get it. I also know that even though all of these things are important, my body does not tolerate this well, so I will need to plan differently in the future. I also know that it means that I need more nutrition, more rest, and more self-care. Yesterday, I had whole-body cryotherapy, local cryo on my face, and red light therapy. I rested, iced, and I am still tired, but my pain is somewhat better today.

I planned a couple of days off of work next week to rest and recover. When we are so far in the red regarding our spoons, we need time to recoup. If my bank account is in the negative, I can't recover that money in a day, I need more time. So, I will take the time that I need to get my spoon bank back in the green. As much as I love Wonder Woman, I am reminded that my titanium does not, in fact, make me invincible. And superheroes also need rest days.

So, my friends, whether you are a spoonie or treating a spoonie, when you are in the red, it takes more than a little rest and recovery. And if you have not had enough self-care to "recharge," your body will tell you so you need to listen. I thought I could keep going and do what I normally do, but I now know that won't suffice for this level of travel.

Follow me for more travel tips. I'm joking but not really. I take everything as a learning experience, and I am learning from this one. My travels have been amazing and hard on my body. My suitcase, for every trip whether it is one night or ten, contains my neck roll, heating pad, lidocaine patches, ice packs, KT tape, tennis balls (to help roll out tight muscles), foot massage ball, and a small foam roller. I also bring a lumbar roll with me to use when I am sitting on the plane. After breaking my wrist and clavicle, I switched to a one-strap laptop bag so I don't have to navigate the airport with a backpack or rolling bag. Hmmm, I am complicated! Yes, I still have plenty of room for my clothes in my bag!

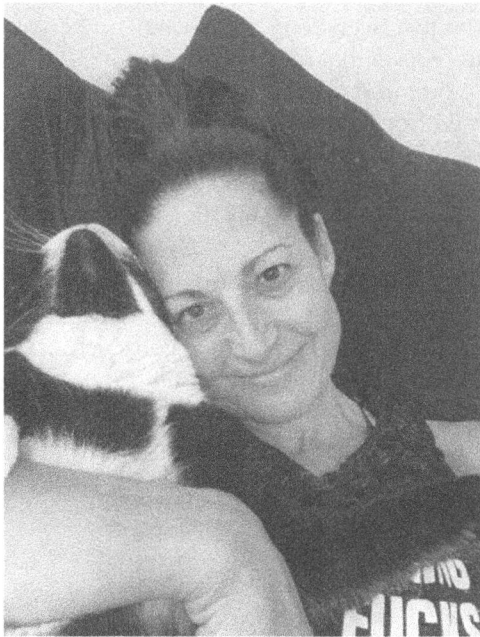

Searching for More Spoons

Think About Cash Flow

Here's another way to look at energy reserves in the frame of money and cash flow. One night, I went to Oregon Dairy with my friend Michelle. It's a cute little Amish market in Lancaster County, Pennsylvania. When we went through the line, I paid with my bank card and tapped to make my payment. I honestly hadn't taken notice of the dollar value of the items in my cart and didn't fully pay attention to the total before I tapped my card. On the other hand, my friend Michelle paid with cash, so she had to be aware of how much she was spending during our little spree. By only having cash on hand, she was more mindful about what she picked up, their dollar value, and even their value to her. She had to consider what was worth her hard-earned cash.

If an individual spends more than they have, they might have a credit card bill that they cannot afford to pay. If a business spends more than it makes, it is in the red, and, eventually, the business will falter because it cannot stay afloat without income.

It is the same with energy reserves. If we spend more than we have and do not take the time to replenish, we can get sick, and it will take a long time to recover. Sometimes, we plan ahead and save some energy in preparation for a big vacation or work trip, just as we would save money for that trip. However, even though we have some energy reserves, there is no guarantee that we won't overspend that money and end up in the red and take a long time to recoup that money/energy.

Individuals may often be driving their energy levels/bank account into the red, possibly without even realizing it. They need to learn how to slow down and work hard at recovering and recouping the money they spent. This can be frustrating because it can be incredibly challenging to make up for overspending. Some days, they might feel as if they have replenished their bank account, only to find that rent is due so that money didn't go far enough. An individual looking to get back into the black should take their time, listen to their body, and take a lesson from my friend Michelle. They should only spend their cash on hand. Sometimes overspending is unavoidable, but individuals should do what they can to stay in the black.

Health Anxiety and Fear of the Future

On top of worrying about and dealing with varied energy levels, individuals with chronic diseases often experience significant anxiety concerning the potential recurrence or worsening of their symptoms. This fear is understandable, as living with long-term conditions can be daunting and overwhelming. The broader concept of *health anxiety* is particularly relevant for individuals navigating these chronic challenges, which can develop slowly and can increase in severity over time. Many chronic diseases are incurable, and treatment typically focuses on managing symptoms rather than achieving a cure. Because of this, patients frequently express feelings of worry and apprehension about their health, which can take an emotional toll.

According to the DSM-5 (diagnostic code 300.7, F45.21), *illness anxiety disorder* is characterized by a deep preoccupation with the fear of having or developing a serious medical condition, even when physical symptoms are absent or mild. This disorder can manifest as either avoidant behavior or a need for constant reassurance. It's important to recognize that a psychiatric diagnosis can now be applied to individuals experiencing excessive health anxiety alongside a diagnosed physical condition, including those living with chronic illnesses. This acknowledgment may provide some comfort to an individual and let them know that they are not alone in their experiences (Cleveland Clinic, 2024).

Most existing research on health anxiety tends to focus on specific illnesses, which can make it challenging for patients to feel understood in their individual struggles. A systematic review of these studies reveals a tendency among researchers to overlook a psychiatric perspective when defining health anxiety and developing theoretical models. Notably, health anxiety affects more than 20 percent of patients in the studies included in this review, highlighting the widespread impact of these fears. While some evidence indicates that health anxiety may remain stable or even decrease over time in certain chronic illnesses, the presence of disability, physical limitations, or noticeable symptoms often serves as a more accurate predictor of health anxiety than objective measures of disease severity.

Understanding one's illness involves navigating multiple dimensions that can be emotionally complex. Patients typically perceive their condition through five key aspects: (a) the believed causes of the illness, (b) their disease label or identity along with the symptoms they associate with that condition, (c) beliefs about the curability or controllability of their illness, (d) anticipated timelines and cyclicality of their situation, and (e) the overall consequences of their condition on their lives. These beliefs significantly influence how individuals cope with their health challenges and the emotional reactions they experience. As a clinician, it's crucial to recognize how difficult it can be for an individual to carry this burden and how these feelings affect both mental and emotional well-being (Lebel et al., 2020).

This systematic review also highlights the maladaptive nature of anxious preoccupation as well as behaviors such as excessive personal checking and over-seeking reassurance from healthcare providers or family members. It's completely natural to feel overwhelmed by these anxieties, especially when faced with the uncertainties of a chronic illness. Acknowledging and addressing these deeply felt fears is not just important; it can be a vital step toward finding comfort and reassurance during such challenging times. It's essential that individuals feel genuinely supported and understood as they navigate their journeys, fostering an environment filled with empathy and compassion where they can express their feelings openly and find solace in the shared experience (Lebel et al., 2020).

Intersection of Spoons, Health Anxiety, and Eating Disorders

Energy levels and health anxiety can also appear in those with eating disorders, with or without a chronic illness. A person with an eating disorder may experience low energy levels due to various factors, such as excessive exercise or malnutrition from food restriction. Additionally, the constant presence of disordered thoughts can take a toll on mental energy. The concept of "lack of spoons" also applies to mental and emotional energy as well as physical energy.

Eating disorders often introduce specific health-related anxieties. Clients typically need to undergo regular medical tests, including lab work, weight checks, and EKGs. Although these tests are necessary, they can trigger anxiety. Clients are educated about the numerous health risks associated with disordered eating, which can further contribute to their health-related worries.

How I Handle Energy Management and Low Moments with Chronic Illness

Not understanding or being able to anticipate energy limits as well as health anxiety can lead to stress and panic about the unknown for individuals. Personally, I try to avoid going down the path of "the sky is falling" with my own chronic illness. I have learned to stay grounded and neutral whenever possible. I am still a human being with fears, and they can occasionally be overwhelming. When we are overwhelmed, it is easy to make assumptions or spiral into negative thinking. We can allow those thoughts to skew our thinking and emotions, and that could lead to a breakdown. A low point does not have to signal disaster, however. An individual can remind themselves that it just means they are out of spoons, have overspent their funds, or are struggling with the chronic nature of their illness. When I run out of spoons, spend more energy than I have, or have a particularly low moment about my scoliosis, I allow myself to feel the consequences and remind myself that I have recovered, will recover, and will figure out how to recharge and reset. Also, I remind myself I don't have to figure it out alone.

Thoughts on Busyness From Someone with a Chronic Medical Condition

September 24, 2020—I've noticed that I've been getting very angry when people tell me that I'm "too busy." During my run, I had a little epiphany, as I often do when I'm running or swimming!

For a long time, I wasn't able to do the things I wanted to do. I wasn't able to visit with friends or go for a run or even sit up for long periods of time without pain. I missed out on a lot of life.

I still struggle with fatigue and have some limitations and some discomfort. However, I am stronger than I've ever been, and **I don't want to miss out on life anymore**. So I want to see my friends and family and have crazy adventures with my swimming and triathlon friends, and enjoy a job that I really love in a career that I am blessed to be a part of.

So I get a little sensitive when people say that I am too busy, as if it is a criticism, because **I fought hard to be busy**. I fought hard for this life and I'm going to live it as much as I can. **There's always a part of me that is afraid of a time where I'm not able to be busy anymore**.

If I have the privilege of being busy, I am going to do it!

Today, a friend of mine and I talked about the concept of the "joy of doing nothing." While I love the concept, I struggle with it because often when I am doing nothing, it is because I am in pain or recovering. It would be a challenge for me to enjoy doing nothing while I actually feel well; however, I think it is worth trying.

Suggestions for Clinicians

Introduce Cognitive Behavioral Therapy and Discuss the Automatic Thought Record

Cognitive behavioral therapy (CBT) is a useful treatment modality for anxiety and other related disorders, and clinicians may find this helpful for individuals with chronic illnesses and eating disorders. CBT is one of my favorite interventions, particularly the exercise of creating an *automatic thought record*. In this approach, the main goal is for an individual to examine their automatic thoughts and feelings. Exercise 13.1 details how to help an individual reframe their thoughts.

For Individuals: How to Understand Your Automatic Thought Record

At times, it can feel like we go from calm to meltdown in 30 seconds. This happens because of the automatic thoughts and feelings that occur as a result of a given situation. For example, if you are experiencing pain from a flare, remember that your physical pain will exacerbate your emotions, so anxiety rated at a 5 without pain might be an 8 with pain. A moment like this requires us to look at the situation, our automatic thoughts, and our feelings as a result of those thoughts, and then we can determine a "hot thought," which is usually one of our core limiting beliefs.

Once we determine those limiting beliefs, we can then decide if those thoughts in the moment are true or not—we do this by looking at evidence for and against these thoughts. Once we have our list of evidence, we then reframe to a more neutral thought and determine our emotions based on that new thought. When we are able to do this, we may still have a meltdown, but it will not feel so automatic or even uncontrollable.

This process takes practice, and it's totally okay to ask for a little help along the way! Your therapist, a friend, or another person in your support team can help you notice and reframe your thoughts. Remember, you're not in this alone, and having someone to lean on can really make a difference.

Exercise 13.1: Help a Client Reframe Their Thoughts

Helping a client develop the skill of reframing their thoughts will change their quality of life. This can help them improve their outlook even if their bodies will never "get better." Reframing thoughts is a choice, and this is one thing that can have an immense impact on someone navigating chronic illness. For example, when I can say to myself, "Just because it hurts, it doesn't mean that I am hurt and that there is something else wrong with me," it reduces my emotions surrounding pain. I can then follow my plan for a pain flare and not react with dread.

To begin this process with your client, walk them through the process of creating an automatic thought record. I have provided the following example from my own life for you to use to describe how this works to a client.

Point out to your clients that this example highlights that the actual situation is not what caused the strong emotions; it was all of the automatic thoughts that created the anxiety and sadness. This example shows that if every time I have additional pain or additional unplanned travel I think that *hot thought* of not being wanted because of my limitations, then I may feel a sense of frustration and sadness.

Sample Automatic Thought Record

Situation	Automatic Thoughts	Feelings (Rate 1-10)	Evidence Supporting	Evidence Against	Neutral Thought	Feelings (Rate 1-10)
I'm on my 3rd day of my new job and, after sitting for 9 hours with 5 hours of driving, I am in intense pain and unable to sleep.	This is never going to get better	Anxious (8)	I have had partners treat me poorly as a result of my limitations	I have many loving friends and the support of my family	Even though I have had negative experiences with employers and partners, I have many friends and supporters who see my value and love me as I am. I have a lot to offer even if I am unable to travel	Anxious (4)
	This is a new pain and I am scared	Sad (6)	I have been left at the hospital, alone, by partners	I have a lot of value, professionally, that is separate from my ability to travel		Sad (3)
	What if I can't do my job because of my limitations	Frustrated (8)	I have had employers discriminate and treat me poorly due to my limitations	My profession spans many different talents, and I will have a plan IF there is a time when I have to limit travel		Frustrated (3)
	There is always a price to pay for doing too much					
	I am not going to be wanted - personally or professionally because of my limitations - HOT THOUGHT					

Figure 13.1 Help a Client Reframe Their Thoughts

Once you have discussed this example with your client, help them create their own automatic thought record by brainstorming situations and working through their automatic thoughts and supporting evidence. Then direct them to come up with neutral thoughts related to these situations to help them reframe their thinking.

Exercise 13.2: Ask Socratic Questions

Another tool to use along with the automatic thought record is asking Socratic questions. These are concise and help to focus on the specific issue you are questioning with your client. These are helpful to use as journal prompts and also to use with your clients in session. There are some great Socratic question worksheets, and you can come up with some specific questions that work best for your client. Some examples of these questions for clients are:

1 Am I basing this thought on facts or feelings?
2 Is this thought black and white when it may be more complicated than that?
3 Am I making assumptions?
4 Is my thought an exaggeration of what is true?
5 Is this thought a habit, or do I have evidence to prove this?
6 Is this thought a worst-case scenario?
7 Could I be misinterpreting the evidence?

Summary

Those with chronic illnesses can share the common language of spoon theory. It helps if clinicians understand this language and can refer to it when discussing pain and energy reserves. In addition to energy reserves, clinicians should consider a client's health anxiety related to their chronic illness and/or eating disorder. DSM-5 offers a diagnosis for illness-related anxiety, or health anxiety. I find CBT most useful when experiencing health anxiety and panic related to a change in prognosis or increased pain. Finding a neutral thought is helpful in processing ongoing illness-related changes and the fear of the future. This can be a useful tool along with spoon theory and considering cash flow for those living with chronic illnesses and eating disorders. In our next chapter, I will examine joyful movement through the lens of chronic medical conditions and eating disorders.

References

About Christine Miserandino. (n.d.). But You Don't Look Sick.com. https://butyou-dontlooksick.com/about/christine-miserandino
Cleveland Clinic. (2024, July 3). Illness Anxiety Disorder (Hypochondria, Hypochondriasis). https://my.clevelandclinic.org/health/diseases/9886-illness-anxiety-disorder-hypochondria-hypochondriasis

Lebel, S., Mutsaers, B., Tomei, C., Leclair, C. S., Jones, G., Petricone-Westwood, D., Rutkowski, N., Ta, V., Trudel, G., Laflamme, S. Z., Lavigne, A.-A., & Dinkel, A. (2020). Health anxiety and illness-related fears across diverse chronic illnesses: A systematic review on conceptualization, measurement, prevalence, course, and correlates. *PLOS ONE, 15*(7). https://doi.org/10.1371/journal.pone.0234124

Natale, G., & Pai, M. (2021). "Spend your spoons wisely": Conceptualizations of time, energy and aging invisibly with Crohn's Disease. *Innovation in Aging, 5*(Supplement_1), 600–601. https://doi.org/10.1093/geroni/igab046.2305

Chapter 14

The Spectrum of Movement: From Fear to Joy

In the field of eating disorders, we work toward intuitive eating as a normal way of life. In recovery, a goal for many is to be able to eat by listening to the body's hunger and fullness signals as well as what type of food they are craving. A similar concept applies to movement; the goal is to find movement that is enjoyable and enhances life. In someone with a chronic medical condition or disability, joyful movement may continue to change over time. There will be times of grief and loss when an individual loses the ability to move in a way that they have come to enjoy, but clinicians can help guide them to reflect on these feelings and find new ways to move that support their bodies and minds.

The Benefits of Movement

Lack of motion can cause an increase in limitations and pain. *Movement* helps every part of our body work in unison—our joints, muscles, and organs. Research shows that movement causes a decrease in pain from conditions such as arthritis. Staying active can be a great way to help manage chronic pain. Many clinical trials have shown that regular exercise can be effective for people dealing with different types of pain. So, getting moving could really make a positive difference for an individual with chronic illness, physically and emotionally (Lima et al., 2017).

My personal experience shows this as well. Even if I am in a period of more limitations (such as the time of this writing as I rest to heal a newly broken big toe), I can still find ways to move my body as well as give it the rest that it needs. Because I tend to be a daredevil and do things "because no one told me not to do them," I ask my medical team to tell me specifically what I can and cannot do. Yes, I do have some fear around injury and pain, but I do not want it to keep me from moving.

The mental health benefits of exercise are well documented. Exercise can prevent and improve various health issues, such as high blood pressure, diabetes, and arthritis. Research indicates that physical activity positively

DOI: 10.4324/9781003500254-19

affects mental health as well, helping to enhance mood and reduce anxiety in individuals suffering from depression and anxiety disorder (Mayo Clinic, 2023).

Considering all of the benefits of movement in individuals with and without chronic illness, a clinician should focus on this aspect of a client's life during treatment.

How Rock Climbing Improves Quality of Life in Patients with Parkinson's Disease

Here's an example of how movement can benefit those with chronic illness. One recent study showed that rock climbing improves symptoms and quality of life in individuals with Parkinson's disease (PD). Researchers observed how a 12-week sport climbing course compared to unsupervised physical training for patients with PD who had never tried climbing before. They discovered two exciting things. First, they found that climbing led to notable improvements in motor symptoms—patients really benefited from it! Second, they learned that climbing is a fun and doable exercise option for PD patients, even if they've never climbed before (Langer et al., 2021).

These positive impacts on those with PD have spurred the creation of rock-climbing programs for those with the condition. Up Ending Parkinson's is a 501(c)(3) nonprofit that provides guided rock climbing for people living with PD. Members have not only found improvement in their movement, they are now a part of a community that supports one another and together they are resilient (Up Ending Parkinsons, 2022). Other programs and resources related to movement and specific chronic illnesses may be available to individuals either locally or through online outlets.

Adaptive Athletes

Up Ending Parkinsons is an example of movement for *adaptive athletes*—people with disabilities who participate or compete in sports with needed modifications or different rules. We see this in the Paralympics and many sports. People commonly think of adaptive athletes as wheelchair basketball players or someone competing in the TCS New York City Marathon using a racing wheelchair. However, differently abled bodies come in all forms, and it may be worth encouraging an individual who has a chronic illness to consider themselves an adaptive athlete and encourage healthy movement and athletic engagement.

Just like anyone else, these athletes can range from novice to amateur to elite athlete. Most sports can be adapted or modified for someone with a disability. We learned about Hope's story in Chapter 12; she is an adaptive athlete who uses a wheelchair. Personally, I have embraced the label of adaptive athlete with my own movement as it relates to my titanium and scoliosis. This helps me set realistic expectations for what my body can do.

Movement as a Way of Life for Those with Eating Disorders and Chronic Illnesses

As clinicians, we want to encourage movement as a way of life, not just as a way to recover from injury or illness. Let's normalize movement in eating disorder recovery and when helping individuals with their chronic illnesses. This has not always been a standard form of treatment and support in eating disorder recovery. Many of us, in early eating disorder recovery, were simply told not to exercise. This was a very confusing direction and had no guideposts, and it vilified all forms of movement and exercise. During treatment, I remember asking myself, "When can I exercise? Is this allowed? Does it mean I've relapsed if I begin moving again?" I had to figure it out on my own and was distraught by the idea of not being allowed to engage in activity because it had benefits for me beyond controlling my body's size.

This is where clinicians and other members of an individual's support team can help someone identify *joyful movement*. What do I mean when I talk about that? This is anything that sparks joy for an individual such as birdwatching, swimming, swinging on rings, or doing anything that makes you smile and feel good in your body. We want individuals to move in an embodied way. To be grounded in their bodies, in the moment, in the movement. It doesn't mean that it isn't challenging; it means that it is something that makes them happy.

What Is "Healthy" Movement?

When discussing *dysfunctional exercise*, it's important to recognize that research has evolved away from traditional metrics like volume, intensity, and frequency. These measures often overlap with the experiences of elite athletes, which can create confusion. Instead, we tend to define dysfunctional exercise through the lens of attitudes, motivations, and beliefs. This can be incredibly nuanced, but some common themes include exercising for appearance, to manage emotions, for identity maintenance, or even as a means of self-harm. Some may find themselves exercising to "earn" food or adhere to strict routines, even if it compromises their physical well-being or safety.

In contrast to the many definitions of dysfunctional exercise, there is much less discussion on what *healthy exercise* looks like, especially in the context of eating disorder recovery and beyond. This gap can leave individuals and clinicians wondering whether it's even possible to achieve a sense of healthy exercise in this journey. It's understandable that differentiating between "healthy" and "dysfunctional" exercise can be quite challenging.

Here's one example of healthy exercise in the context of weightlifting. One illuminating study focused on women in eating disorder recovery who took up weightlifting (Hockin-Boyers & Warin, 2021). These women were not elite athletes, but they found something special in the structured nature of weightlifting that offered them feelings of "calm" and "safety." It provided them with a way to compartmentalize exercise within the hectic pace of daily life. For these participants, the need for structure became a source of support and well-being. Weightlifting prompted a shift in their mindset—from focusing on appearance to embracing personal challenges. Through the lens of "gains," they began to see food and eating as something that honored their bodies rather than working against them.

Interestingly, many participants mentioned that other forms of exercise, like yoga, running, or dance, didn't provide them with the same level of confidence and acceptance in embracing their bodies. They shared that "healthy" exercise should promote feelings of strength, joy, and a reduction in stress. It's heartening to see that they are finding paths that resonate with their needs and support their journey toward self-acceptance and well-being (Hockin-Boyers & Warin, 2021).

No Type of Exercise Is Inherently Bad for Chronic Illnesses and Eating Disorders

Exercise for someone with an eating disorder or chronic illness is not inherently bad. While it can be misused and become an issue, we cannot assume that any movement that someone with an eating disorder practices is disordered. We also must stop pathologizing certain types of movement such as running. There is a common assumption that if you are a runner, you are orthorexic or disordered, and that is just not true. We need to be careful with any generalizations like this. No sport or movement is inherently bad. Yes, we do know that there are some sports that can predispose someone to the development of an eating disorder, and yet it is also true that someone can return to sport, with the support of a treatment team, in a healthy way.

Movement for those with chronic illness may be similarly confusing if individuals have to modify their exercise routines because of a diagnosis, pain, or other new symptoms. Just as with individuals with eating disorders, it is important that an individual with a chronic illness identify healthy ways to move their body that do not impact their condition negatively. It is important for clinicians to frame the benefits of certain kinds of movement for those with eating disorders and chronic illnesses and not treat physical activity as a restricted or all-or-nothing game.

Fear of Movement

Many individuals face a deep-seated fear of movement, especially when linked to specific health conditions. They may have been injured or experienced negative consequences of moving their bodies in certain ways because of chronic illness and/or an eating disorder and have developed mental and physical blocks that prevent them from finding healthy ways to move. A clinician should try to understand an individual's fear of movement to help them work through their complicated emotions surrounding physical activity.

One study highlighted the emotional struggle some individuals experience when it comes to cardiovascular exercise, revealing that this fear can lead to poorer outcomes in cardiac and pulmonary rehabilitation. It's completely understandable that anxiety about uncomfortable physical sensations may arise, making it difficult to engage in exercise. Many individuals find themselves grappling with these fears and often try to avoid physical activity altogether. In pulmonary rehabilitation, this avoidance is not just a physical challenge; it also correlates with increased levels of anxiety and depression. It's important for individuals to acknowledge these feelings and work toward a supportive environment that encourages movement and healing (Farris et al., 2019).

One study examined fear of movement as it relates to back and neck pain. Fear avoidance is a common response many people experience when dealing with pain. It can feel natural to believe that avoiding movement or activity will help reduce pain or prevent further injury. This fear often stems from past experiences of pain, leading to a cycle where individuals shy away from activities they believe might cause discomfort, including physical exercise (Jadhakhan et al., 2022).

Movement avoidance can significantly impact daily life, making it more difficult to engage in activities that once brought joy or fulfillment. It can also lead to social isolation such as canceling plans that include physical activities such as a walk or a hike. It's understandable that if an individual is living with spinal pain, they may find themselves worried about the possibility of worsening their condition. However, research shows that these fears and beliefs about movement can lead to negative outcomes, including the development of physical disabilities (Jadhakhan et al., 2022).

Exploring Resistance to Exercise

June 2024—This week I had the honor of being a presenter on a webinar for the International Scientific Scoliosis Association. I presented about scoliosis, spine fusion, and resilience. We discussed many topics including inactivity. A conversation about movement would be incomplete without a discussion about inactivity and exercise resistance.

What we know is that inactivity can lead to increased pain, stiffness, and limitations. This exercise resistance can come from many areas, and it is important to explore where that stems from and address that. We cannot suggest a solution without examining the underlying cause. For example, someone may have had a negative experience with physical therapy in the past or they may have had a harsh baseball coach. Any negative past experiences with movement can lead to a fear of movement and resistance to exercise in any form.

authortamiegangloff

Scoliosis, Spine Fusion and Resilience

척추측만증, 척추 융합 및 회복력

Tamie Gangloff MA HFT
USA

View insights   Boost post

♡ 20   ◯ 2   ▽ 2

Liked by ___ nd others
authortamiegangloff It was such an honor to be a part of this webinar this morning to talk to physiotherapists in South Korea, about scoliosis, spine fusion... more
___ Thank you for your valuable announcement early in the morning ^^ I will try to have continuous exchange in the future. Good night.

Exploring Resistance to Exercise

Pushing Past Exercise Aversion or Resistance

Some individuals may develop an *aversion or resistance to exercise* based on a past negative experience. For some clients, this means that they will not return to a sport that they love, or they may not partake in any movement at all whether that is walking or going to the gym.

I had a former client who was asked to leave their high school swim team due to an eating disorder. It was devastating, and this was a traumatic experience for them, so they developed exercise resistance. *Exercise resistance* can be interpreted in many ways; to me, it means that someone is not willing or able to exercise out of fear, anxiety, or trauma surrounding exercise. This is not very different from an athlete who has experienced a severe injury and has a fear of returning to sport. With this client, for one of our therapy sessions, we met at the pool to experience wearing a swimsuit and getting into the water. They chose to get in the water and swim a little, and they experienced joy in the water for the first time in many years. This was such an important step in moving past their trauma, anxiety, and struggle to get in the water again. Today, they continue to swim with joy.

Profile: How Eating Disorder Treatment Confused Her Relationship with Exercise

In someone with an eating disorder, there is another aspect to the story of healthy movement. I recently interviewed my friend Ella about her experience. She said:

> I was always super active, as a kid, and was always heavily involved in gymnastics and cheer for many hours per week. Through my eating disorder, I never struggled with overexercise or saw it as a negative thing. At that time, if I didn't feel well, I didn't force myself to exercise, I would rest. As time went on and I was in my eating disorder longer, I would go to practice and perform. I did not see it as a negative until I went into treatment for my eating disorder, and I then developed the idea that exercise was bad. It seemed as if all exercise was demonized and assumed to be a part of the eating disorder. Later on, I learned that movement is actually helpful for me.

Ella continued:

> I feel like eating disorder treatment "messed up" my relationship with exercise more than my eating disorder itself did. Also, while I was in treatment, I discovered that exercise reconnected me with my physical self. I feel like a "floating head" but when I incorporate movement, I reconnect those two pieces and it can be jarring but also grounding. It can feel really uncomfortable, but it is really helpful.

Embodiment

Ella's story perfectly describes an important concept of movement for everyone, and particularly those with eating disorders and/or chronic illnesses: *embodiment*. This is when someone is fully present in the moment, in their body, grounded in movement. Framing movement as an aspect of embodiment may be a helpful way to treat individuals with fear of movement and confusion about exercise and other physical activities as a result of their eating disorder and/or chronic illness.

My dear friend and fellow clinician Johanna Kulp just published her book *Finding Peace with Your Body: A Guide for All Women*. She describes embodiment in the following way:

> Embodiment is the opposite of the silence we held on to in our criticalness and judgment. In being embodied we are so involved and connected to our bodies that we let them guide us. As stated before, we first work through our thoughts as we heal our body image. But full healing brings our mind and our bodies back together, connecting both in a way that creates not only a relationship but a togetherness. Embodiment is all about empathy at its core. We can't BE IN our body without also having a level of compassion for it.
>
> (Kulp, 2025)

Embodiment is a way for individuals to hold empathy but not pity for their bodies, as Kulp further describes:

> If we don't feel the empathy and compassion for it, we are constantly at odds, fighting with it rather than living in it. I want to be careful here: Empathy does not denote some level of pity or sadness. In fact, when I have empathy and embodiment, I feel proud of my thighs and proud of my body. I move past neutrality into pride for myself and my body. Beyond just rebuilding, embodiment is reconnecting so that we can feel tangibly connected and close to our bodies again. It's a reconnection so that our mind and body are once again together. It's a reconnection so that while we are walking, running, gardening, or doing whatever else with our bodies, we are simply IN our bodies, not scrutinizing or judging. **You can be embodied, fully present and involved in your body.**
>
> (Kulp, 2025)

Feeling empathy toward one's body allows individuals to move past fear, anger, and frustration with movement as the result of their eating disorder and/or chronic illness. Personally, I have experienced going to physical therapy feeling frustrated with my body. If I can reframe the situation through the lens of empathy and listen to my body with understanding and kindness, I can then move toward understanding and acceptance. With empathy, we can allow ourselves grace and that will then make space for finding a solution, whether that is searching for new movement, finding new meaning, or asking for more help.

Managing Fear with Chronic Illness and Eating Disorder Symptoms

Individuals with chronic illnesses and/or eating disorders may struggle with embodiment because by being fully in their body, they may be concerned that they will be subject to all of the symptoms of their conditions. However, I would argue that feeling what's inside of one's body is a way for someone to better understand their abilities and limitations and make choices that correspond to what their body can tolerate.

Take, for example, pain and fear of pain. There are ways we can work on managing pain and anxiety around pain, and fear of the pain is often worse than the pain itself. This is where embodiment can help an individual recognize their body's signals. Without them, we don't know when we need to see a doctor, get an x ray, or pull a wrist brace out of the drawer for a bit until the pain gets better. Having a high tolerance for pain and other bothersome symptoms and circumstances surrounding a chronic illness or eating disorder isn't always a good thing because it means that an individual can miss out on important signals from their body. The more an individual ignores, the more they risk further injury or illness and miss out on the awesome sensations in life! This is where embodiment could help them move past pain and get professional help to relieve symptoms.

For someone with an eating disorder, this becomes even more complicated. There are so many layers here. An individual might worry that they will feel hunger, fullness, bloating, anxiety, anger, or other physical sensations that are oftentimes unbearable. They may have been fighting these feelings for years, and reintroducing them into their life could seem cruel, like an impossible and unfair ask. However, part of recovery is gaining the ability to tolerate these sensations and then learning to accept them and embrace them as a part of who we are. Instead of the fear that might come from feeling hungry and full, an individual might welcome it as they have dinner plans with friends and want to enjoy food with them. Keep in mind that this is not an automatic process and may take many years of work for an individual to get to this place of embodiment.

Broken Bones and Reconnecting with Our Bodies

Last year, I broke some bones racing, and my body is still recovering. My body keeps telling me this in many ways, such as with bruises and a sprained thumb and wrist from doing a movement that typically would not cause this. My body is saying "knock it off." I have had to adjust how I move my body following this injury. While I really love obstacle course racing, I have decided that I will no longer race, even though I love my team and the training. But just because I can flip a tire doesn't mean I should. So it is time for me to do something different again. This is a hard shift to accept, but I can feel this in my core. I experienced grief related to the decision, but after some time, I feel at peace and am able to turn to my intuition for solutions. This is something I could not do without being grounded and embodied.

To be clear, there are times when we are not fully in our bodies or fully embodied. Sometimes this is self-preservation and typically it is an unconscious choice. Living alone through my broken-bone era, there were some layers of disconnection I had to feel, from my body, in order to function with day-to-day tasks such as washing my hair and changing my sheets. It was not a conscious choice, but I had to keep moving and taking care of myself, my home, and my cats. This translates to other areas of life as well.

Spectrum of Joyful Movement

Does movement *have* to be joyful? Absolutely not! As clinicians, we would like it to spark joy for our clients, of course. It would be great if we could find joy in the moment even if we can't find it in the movement. For example, physical therapy is often painful, but if I can chat or laugh with the PTs or PTAs, then it can bring some enjoyment. Sometimes I am bored at the gym, so it doesn't spark joy, while I know that it is important to stay strong at the same time. Maybe the choice of workout music can spark some joy even when the movement itself might not bring joy.

I want to make this distinction because, for many people, movement is not joyful. It might be more helpful to look at movement on a spectrum; it is fluid and can be painful to neutral to joyful. Fluidity is important. If an individual is in a chronically ill body, they will likely experience all of these feelings, and they will continue to shift and change. For example, as I write this today, my goal is to do some strength training and stretching. My neck is hurting quite a bit, so I will not do some of the things I enjoy because they might irritate my body more. I might find some joy in my workout, but it is more specifically neutral movement. It will "get the job done" by giving my body what it needs, even though it might not spark the same joy I feel when I am in the open water, running with friends, or swinging on the rings.

Suggestions for Clinicians on Treating Exercise and Movement

How to Address Fear of Movement

Someone with a chronic medical condition may have a fear of exercise, a valid fear. Whether they grew up being told not to exercise or they are fearful of getting hurt, they may stay away from exercise out of this concern.

We know that movement is medicine and that even though one's abilities may change over time, we can adapt movement so it is joyful.

Your client may need to devise a plan that relies on the support of many as they determine what healthy movement means for their own situation. They can:

- Work with a compassionate and knowledgeable physical therapist who may alleviate fear of doing something that might hurt them.
- Hire a coach or personal trainer skilled in working with a disability who can walk them through their fears.
- Try exposure therapy with a friend or coach to help them slowly expose themselves to their fears.
- Work out with teammates; they can do their PT while they work out so there is still togetherness and support even if they can't engage in all of the activities.
- Utilize EMDR if the valid fear is due to a trauma such as an accident during working out or racing.
- Ask for modifications and support to get their needs met.

Exercises for Clinicians

Exercise 14.1: Ask Questions About Your Client's Experiences with Movement

Let's first get curious and ask questions. We learn about our patients through their stories, so we must learn those before we can offer support. Our goal is to help our patients discover joyful movement; still, we may have many steps to take before we can get there.

Ask your client the following questions to begin:

1 Can you remember a time when you enjoyed movement?
2 What was it?
3 How old were you?
4 How did it feel? Be as descriptive as possible.

Then ask them about the unpleasant or traumatic experiences as well:

1 Were your parents strict about exercise?
2 Did you have a tough coach?
3 Did you have to perform through pain?

Once we have brainstormed what movement is joyful with the client, let's also make sure that it is recommended by medical providers, whether that is a physical therapist or physician. With your client, come up with a plan and steps to get there. This is another time where SMART goals can be useful.

Exercise 14.2: Administer the Exercise Dependence Scale

Exercise dependence is a complex issue that often doesn't occur on its own; it frequently exists alongside eating disorders or body dysmorphic disorder. Many individuals facing these challenges may find themselves in a cycle where exercise becomes a source of stress rather than stress relief.

The Exercise Dependence Scale, consisting of 30 thoughtful questions, serves as a tool to help assess the level of tolerance and addiction associated with exercise. It encourages reflection on important questions, such as whether someone can take a break from exercising for health reasons or whether they might push through pain from an injury to continue their routine.

It's crucial to recognize that exercise dependence can lead to excessive and obsessive behaviors, ultimately resulting in physical injuries or health issues (Adams, 2013). If you suspect that your client is struggling with exercise dependence, I recommend utilizing this scale.

This can show up differently in someone with a chronic medical condition. They may be used to functioning at a high level of pain which makes it possible to continue to exercise or compete in the presence of pain and injury.

Exercise 14.3: Questions for Eating Disorder Recovered Athletes

Once recovered from an eating disorder, many who struggled have gone on to become triathletes, marathon runners, obstacle course racers, long distance swimmers, and the list goes on. Clients can do this as long as they are listening to their bodies and nourishing themselves.

Before engaging in sport, we need to ask our client important questions:

1 Are you nourishing your body for movement? (Please enlist the support of your registered dietician.)
2 Are you taking rest days?
3 How do you feel in your body and mind when you move?
4 How do you feel emotionally if you need to take an extra rest day due to travel or illness?
5 Are you able to be flexible with your workout plans if you need to change days and times?

Exercise 14.4: Activities for Clients to Connect with Their Bodies

Here are some activities for clients to use to connect with their bodies. These will help them slow down and engage in centering practices. You may want to go over these options and instruct them on any activities that sound appealing to them.

• Practice grounding with the five senses
• Eat mindfully
• Drink something cold

- Journal about feelings
- Check in with a trusted friend, sponsor, family member
- Spend time in nature
- Spend time with pets or animals
- Check in with your hunger and fullness
- Practice grounding breaths

Summary

Research indicates that movement is beneficial both physically and emotionally. When dealing with chronic illness and eating disorders, it is important to approach movement with caution and intention. Sometimes movement can be a joyful experience, while at other times it may be necessary for rehabilitation after an injury. For those recovering from an eating disorder, returning to sport is achievable, provided they plan ahead, have support, and engage in movement that feels embodied. A fear of movement can be a significant barrier, but it is possible to overcome this fear and move forward in recovery. As clinicians, we must be careful not to demonize exercise or instill a fear of movement in our clients. It is essential to meet our clients where they are and create opportunities for them to engage in movement that is healthy and grounded in their bodies. In the next chapter, we will explore the impact of chronic illness on relationships.

References

Adams, J. (2013). Exercise Dependence—an Overview. ScienceDirect. www.sciencedirect.com/topics/psychology/exercise-dependence

Farris, S. G., Abrantes, A. M., Bond, D. S., Stabile, L. M., & Wu, W.-C. (2019). Anxiety and fear of exercise in cardiopulmonary rehabilitation. *Journal of Cardiopulmonary Rehabilitation and Prevention, 39*(2), E9–E13. https://doi.org/10.1097/hcr.0000000000000401

Hockin-Boyers, H., & Warin, M. (2021). Women, exercise, and eating disorder recovery: The normal and the pathological. *Qualitative Health Research, 31*(6), 104973232199204. https://doi.org/10.1177/1049732321992042

Jadhakhan, F., Sobeih, R., & Falla, D. (2022). Effects of exercise/physical activity on fear of movement in people with spine-related pain: Protocol for a systematic review and meta-analysis. *BMJ Open, 12*(5), e060264. https://doi.org/10.1136/bmjopen-2021-060264

Kulp, J. (2025). *Finding Peace with Your Body: A Body Image Guide for Women.* Routledge.

Langer, A., Hasenauer, S., Flotz, A., Gassner, L., Pokan, R., Dabnichki, P., Wizany, L., Gruber, J., Roth, D., Zimmel, S., Treven, M., Schmoeger, M., Willinger, U., Maetzler, W., & Zach, H. (2021). A randomised controlled trial on effectiveness and feasibility of sport climbing in Parkinson's disease. *npj Parkinson's Disease, 7*(1), 1–9. https://doi.org/10.1038/s41531-021-00193-8

Lima, L. V., Abner, T. S. S., & Sluka, K. A. (2017). Does exercise increase or decrease pain? Central mechanisms underlying these two phenomena. *The Journal of Physiology, 595*(13), 4141–4150. https://doi.org/10.1113/jp273355

Mayo Clinic. (2023, December 23). Depression and anxiety: Exercise eases symptoms. www.mayoclinic.org/diseases-conditions/depression/in-depth/depression-and-exercise/art-20046495

Up Ending Parkinsons. (2022). Who we are. www.upendingparkinsons.org/?ftag=MSF0951a18

Chapter 15

Impact of Chronic Illness on Relationships

In eating disorder recovery, we often hear from clients that when they *looked sick*, they received the love and support that they didn't feel capable of asking for. In treatment, we work with clients on the skill of being able to ask to get their needs met no matter what their symptoms.

In addition, someone with a chronic illness may have visible or invisible symptoms, and they may question when it is appropriate to ask for help. They may think they must look or be sick to feel loved and supported. In this chapter, we will unpack these beliefs and how an individual can ask for support for both their physical and emotional needs from a place of vulnerability that does not require active symptoms from their chronic illness or eating disorder.

I do feel that many individuals are suffering in silence, only reaching out to support systems when absolutely necessary. Recently, I had to go to urgent care, and I was nervous. Part of me thought that I should call a friend to see if they could take me or meet me there. Then I thought, "Nah, it's too much trouble, I'll just go alone." As I write this, I am reminded of what I said at the Root to Branch gala some time ago: "No one should ever sit at urgent care or the emergency room alone. If you need someone to go with you, call me." I have sat alone, and I never want anyone to have to experience that. I am hopeful this chapter will advocate for individuals to identify and foster relationships that provide support and love as they navigate chronic illnesses, eating disorders, and other challenges.

Chronic Illness and Relationships

Impact of Chronic Illness on Relationships

Having a disability of any kind, whether it is physical or mental, can have an impact on an individual's relationships. These include an individual's:

- Family of origin
- Friendships

DOI: 10.4324/9781003500254-20

- Chosen family
- Employer
- Romantic partnerships
- Recovery community

In ideal partnerships, individuals share burdens, good times, and difficult times. Often, a disability is a third party in a relationship.

We-ness and Communal Coping

Communal coping is a relational approach where a couple collectively perceives a problem or medical condition as a shared challenge—framing it as "our" issue instead of attributing it to just one partner. This perspective fosters cooperation and mutual support, allowing both individuals to work together to address the situation and strengthen their bond in the process.

In a study exploring the experiences of couples facing heart failure, researchers uncovered an important insight: when a spouse or partner expressed "we talk," it was linked to positive changes in the patient's health outcomes. This groundbreaking research highlights the significant role that supportive communication can play in navigating chronic illness together, emphasizing how the use of the "we" pronoun can foster better understanding and connection between partners during challenging times (Rohrbaugh, 2020).

Zephyr and Agamemnon's Story: A Sick Love Story

Trigger warning: this story contains detailed information about eating disorders and triggers as well as chronic illness.

Zephyr and Agamemnon are a couple who have been witness to each other's chronic illnesses and eating disorders, and who have learned to support each other through it all. They have an amazing love story, made even more awe-inspiring by their passion for supporting one another regardless of ability or adversity. Together they are a force.

Both Zephyr and Agamemnon are eating disorder clinicians who are well known in the field. I first saw Zephyr, who specializes in art therapy and identifies as fat, nonbinary, queer, and disabled, present at an eating disorder conference and was immediately a fangirl. They wore a sequin bodysuit with a decked-out cane. They were powerful, confident, and authentic. Agamemnon, also an art therapist, is an extraordinary clinician, has an incredible sense of humor, and loves fiercely. He specializes in sexuality, gender, and body image.

Zephyr and Agamemnon met in 2010 on OK Cupid on the internet and, after several months of chatting, became "Facebook official." About six months later, they moved in together and then got engaged. Since that time, they have battled through medical minefields and eating disorder treatments, learning many valuable lessons along the way.

Individual Histories of Eating Disorders and Chronic Illness

Before Zephyr met Agamemnon, they lived with an eating disorder that was based on restriction and overexercise. This was the result of doctors telling Zephyr to lose weight because of other symptoms of a disability, which at that time was undiagnosed. "They [doctors] tell you to lose weight and it will get better so you do it and then it makes the disability worse." Zephyr also held on to baggage from their childhood related to disability.

Zephyr tried to manage chronic pain with their weight management and held on to fears about chronic illness based on her childhood. Their mother had polio as a child and would speak of cruel and painful treatments. However, because of the culture, she did not admit to a disability, though she did have a significant limp. She wouldn't use a mobility aid or get a handicap placard. So as Zephyr began to have their own experience, they knew that they did not want to feel tortured like their mom was.

Agamemnon also carried eating-related issues to their relationship. Looking back, Agamemnon wasn't overweight as a kid. He didn't grow up with a lot of money, so he was in the "clean plate club" and was taught the "are you sure you want to do that [eat that]" mentality. His family had limited resources, and there was some food insecurity in his home. Agamemnon started experiencing disordered eating in college after breaking up with his girlfriend and moving back home. He would go to the gym when his family sat down for dinner, and he would be there for hours. He didn't take days off—every day was leg day, every day was ab day—it didn't matter what day it was. He was also eating much less than the recommended calories per day, and he lost the weight quickly. He knew that was not sustainable.

Agamemnon grew up with a mom who had multiple sclerosis but, like Zephyr's mom, never treated it as a disability. Growing up, he saw her take her medication, and sometimes she was tired, but there was little discussion about her well-being. He and his dad took his mom to medical appointments because they only had one car, but this was viewed more as a family activity than something they "had" to do.

Disordered Eating as a Couple

When Zephyr and Agamemnon got together, they were both in a disordered eating cycle. They would binge weekends because they "earned" it. They would wake up at 4:30 a.m. to make it to the gym by 5 a.m. They were young, aspiring graduate students who had little money, which can often lead to certain food choices because of food insecurity. (They have vowed to never again have those awful 100-calorie soups or a gym membership.) By the time they were halfway through grad school, their disordered eating had improved, other than going a little too hard at the gym sometimes.

First Signs of Illness

Right before their engagement trip to Scotland, Zephyr had their first set of MRIs, x-rays, and ultrasounds because they were having trouble walking after going out dancing. They woke up to everything hurting—everything from their hips down was swollen, their joints hurt, and they thought they must have injured themself when dancing, or that maybe they had worn the wrong shoes. Zephyr was told that there was nothing wrong with them and they just needed to lose some weight. For someone in recovery, hearing that was damaging.

Zephyr had a thorough and caring primary care doctor, and they sat with them for over two hours and went over every test, every symptom, and their entire history. Even though they didn't have a definitive diagnosis, they agreed to call it fibromyalgia to start medication and physical therapy. Zephyr blamed themselves. "I'm in a bigger body, I had bariatric surgery, I guess I should be in pain." Their doctor countered this harmful line of thinking, saying that no one would cause this to themselves.

Weight Loss Surgery

Zephyr decided to undergo bariatric surgery following this diagnosis because weight loss was suggested, as it is for many health conditions. Bariatric surgeons need to screen for eating disorders, but many are not thorough. Zephyr did the EDE-Q© (Eating Disorder Examination Questionnaire) at home without a therapist. At this time, they were a few years from becoming a licensed therapist, but they were working in the eating disorder field and were very knowledgeable. Despite self-administering the exam, no one within the surgical team looked into how this procedure might affect Zephyr's eating disorder history. No one talked to Zephyr's therapist. Zephyr told the medical team that they were in recovery, but they weren't in the "right" recovery. They met with a social worker and a movement specialist who showed them how to move if you are "too fat" to move. There were a lot of beige flags. But Zephyr just wanted to feel better so badly that they ignored them.

Zephyr had the surgery and lost the weight, but they started to become vitamin deficient. Their disability got worse instead of better; movement got harder instead of easier. The recovery triggered a lot of Zephyr's eating disorder history, including strict rules for eating (American Society for Metabolic and Bariatric Surgery, n.d.).

Ultimately, the surgery did nothing to help Zephyr's symptoms, and they often wonder what their life and disability would look like if they had never had the surgery.

What If This is Too Much for You?

Before and after this procedure, Zephyr experienced debilitating symptoms from their chronic illness. Zephyr would say to Agamemnon, "I totally understand if this is too much for you." He always rebuffs them after this comment. Agamemnon takes Zephyr to all of their appointments, and when he can't be there, he will call Zephyr's dad and ask if he will go with them. When asked how they accept the love and support, Zephyr responded, "I don't have a choice—Agamemnon is very good at saying that I know that this is uncomfortable and get in the car."

Zephyr and Agamemnon joke that "Waiting Room" by Fugazi is his anthem (seriously, look up the lyrics). He does not have a problem waiting outside appointments as long as he has something to do. He can get annoyed when appointments take much longer than expected, but he is annoyed at the medical system, not at Zephyr.

Mobility Aids

Both Agamemnon and Zephyr use mobility aids. Agamemnon sometimes uses a cane for a herniated disc, but he has difficulty considering using a wheelchair for himself. Zephyr has overcome the hesitation of using a wheelchair, but they do struggle if someone has to push them. They had an experience where Agamemnon had to push a wheelchair up a gravel path. They had even called ahead to make sure the path was disability friendly; however, it was not. "When you are in a bigger body going up a hill, that is a lot to ask of someone." It was the most terrible experience they have had mobility-wise ever.

Because of his professional training, Agamemnon is able to address some of the elephants in the room about disabilities and intimacy. For instance, he talks about shower chairs. "In every movie where you see a couple taking a shower, there is not a shower chair in the shower. Most movies about a disability are depressing and inaccurate. People are so uncomfortable talking about sex in that capacity." But Ron points out that the shower chair can lead to intimacy in the shower rather than symbolize something that a person can't do.

Agamemnon pushes through his health symptoms because Zephyr experiences more severe symptoms from their chronic illness. If two people are chronically ill or disabled, whoever is in more pain "wins" that day, meaning they are the one that gets taken care of.

They also have worked through a lot of issues related to trust because of these health issues. Zephyr struggles that Agamemnon or someone else needs to push them in their wheelchair and they must provide feedback if something doesn't feel right in the chair. "If something doesn't feel right in the chair, I must tell him, and I can't see what he sees. We've had arguments and he had said, 'You have to trust me.' It takes time, therapy, fighting, and all of the normal things that people go through. It is just different when it is about what your body can and cannot do in the world."

Attachment Trauma and Chronic Illness

Attachment trauma is a deeply painful experience that occurs when there is a significant disruption in the bond between a caregiver and their child. This disruption may take many forms, often stemming from an absence of nurturing, care, and reliable support during crucial developmental moments. Understanding this can help us recognize its profound impact on a child's emotional well-being and the importance of fostering healthy connections for healing and growth. (Attachment Project, n.d.)

We call this an attachment wound or an attachment injury in adult relationships. It is a painful disruption in an intimate relationship that can arise from feelings of betrayal or abandonment. This experience can be deeply unsettling, often touching on our core emotions and vulnerabilities. It is important to understand how this relates to attachment trauma, which involves ongoing interruptions in the bonds we form in childhood. While attachment trauma manifests as a series of distressing experiences over time, an attachment wound typically results from a single, significant event. Recognizing and addressing these feelings can be crucial to healing and rebuilding trust in our relationships (Attachment Project, 2023).

Clinicians must recognize that individuals with chronic illnesses may not always have loving, supportive relationships to help them manage their symptoms. Many who have chronic medical conditions struggle in relationships. Sometimes an individual suffers consequences for their limitations, and relationship struggles are part of their normal. The price that someone pays in these problematic relationships can include their dignity, safety, financial security, friendships, and emotional and spiritual well-being.

For example, prior to my spinal fusion in 2018, and for some time after, I was in a narcissistic, abusive relationship. It wasn't until I discovered new life after my surgery and months-long recovery that I found the courage to leave the relationship. It is never easy to get out of an abusive relationship and even more daunting and frightening when one has physical limitations.

This is another reason why a group support is vital. In eating disorder and chronic illness support groups, peers get to help one another and know that they are not alone in navigating life and relationships while recovering from their eating disorder and living in a differently abled body.

Dating with a Chronic Illness

Dating can be especially challenging for those individuals who have chronic illnesses as well as eating disorders. As blogger Ellen Davidson states in her article "A Sick Girl's Guide to Navigating Dating with a Chronic Illness," "the harsh reality is not everyone is willing to date someone with a chronic condition."

I have experienced the challenges of dating with a chronic illness firsthand. Finding a romantic partner has been made even more difficult because of my sobriety. When I used dating apps, I struggled to decide when to disclose both my spine fusion and my sobriety, but I often decided to get it out into the open early. While anyone can get sick at any point in a relationship, how much does a stranger want or need to know about an individual's health? I often felt the need to justify myself following these disclosures—for instance, stating, "I am cool if you drink; it doesn't bother me to be around alcohol" or "I am healthy and strong and very active so my spine is not an issue." *These were sales pitches that I was not too defective to date.* Rejection never feels good, but I wanted people to have the information upfront so they could move on from me early on instead of later if these were deal-breakers. Some potential dates have ghosted me after they had that information or "changed their mind" and stated that they are only looking for something casual.

Being single and experiencing or anticipating rejection can take a toll on one's well-being. For example, despite my full life with an amazing career, friends, family, and relative health, I struggle in romantic partnerships and meeting potential companions. Do I blame my spine? Definitely not, but it is a factor. I have done therapy including EMDR and I continue to work on this (Davidson, 2024).

I do know that my limitations have been held against me in relationships. So, I carry that fear with me into dating and potential new relationships. In some ways, I wear it as if it were armor, protecting myself with it. *See, I am single because no one wants to deal with me and my medical issues …* This is an example of *confirmation bias*, which means that an individual is looking for information that confirms what they already believe to be true.

Over time, my perspective on dating has shifted. I found solace in what Gladwell (2020) writes: "I realized that if someone couldn't be with me because I have a chronic health condition, it wasn't a relationship I needed." I would love to see more written about chronic illness and romantic relationships. Currently, there are only a few articles out there on this topic without a lot of research available.

Friendships with a Chronic Illness

Friendships can be a meaningful source of support for those with chronic illness, and they don't have to be that different from what an individual would get from a romantic partner. One can find love, help, and vulnerability in their friendships, though friends may not be part of an individual's daily life like a romantic partner. This physical distance may require an individual to be more clear about their needs with their friends.

In my own life, my friends and family showed up when I broke my bones in 2023. They opened Gatorade bottles, took me grocery shopping, put my hair in a ponytail, picked up my fat cat, and helped me clean. They texted me every day to see how I was feeling. They love me for all of me with scars and titanium; they might even love me more for it.

Being Single with a Chronic Illness

The other day, a family member asked me if it was better to be single than in a relationship. And I answered by saying that there are a lot of good things about being single. I can choose my life, make my own choices, buy myself presents! I told her that it can be challenging, such as living alone through my broken bones or sometimes just needing a hug to feel better.

Creating a life as a single person with a disability is unique. A single person can still enjoy all of the perks of being single, but they also need to ask for help and plan ahead. It is possible to figure out anything, but sometimes an individual's emotional state can make it difficult to see the solution. Plan ahead for help. Reach out to others to ask for help in finding solutions.

Strategies for Single Living

Here are some of the tips I share for individuals living alone with a chronic illness. I understand that everyone has different financial resources available to them, so some of these recommendations may not be relevant.

Get Help with Cleaning

Hire a cleaning service, ask a friend for help, or utilize free cleaning and cooking services offered in some communities for those with disabilities.

Find Easier Ways to Feed Yourself

Cooking and meal prep have never been my favorite activities, and this can be particularly challenging for anyone who is single. Who really enjoys cooking for just one person? Fortunately, there are many options available: meal prep services, meal delivery, grocery delivery, and even asking for help from friends. For instance, when I broke my wrist, several friends accompanied me on grocery shopping trips and offered assistance.

One effective strategy is to prepare meals in larger quantities to have leftovers that can last for several days or be frozen for future use. It's perfectly okay if you don't aspire to be like Martha Stewart and whip up elaborate meals for one. It's okay to rely on convenience foods and a variety of snacks to simplify things. Convenience foods often receive a bad reputation for not being as "healthy" as home-cooked meals. However, it is better to eat something convenient rather than skipping a meal altogether. There's a lot of stigma and judgment regarding prepared foods, and nobody needs to encounter that.

I'm fortunate to have some great markets nearby, so sometimes I pick up "home-cooked" meals prepared by wonderful local vendors. Additionally, when I'm in pain, it's tough to eat a full meal, so I often opt for many smaller meals and snacks throughout the day. Ordering groceries online is also a great option!

Consider Transportation Options

Reach out to go-to people to ask for a ride for appointments. This will also provide moral support and hopefully some levity and laughs. If this is not possible, schedule an Uber or Lyft. These can be a bit pricey, so if this is a regular need, see if there are services in the area that provide transportation for those with disabilities.

Actionable Steps for Clinicians

Determine Relationship Patterns

If you are a therapist working with a client who has a chronic illness, it's important to pay attention to their relationship patterns. Ask relevant questions, as clients may feel like they have to face negative consequences for needing help. I know I felt that way myself. Consequently, your client might not recognize that their relationships are unhealthy.

Focus on Solution-Focused Couples Therapy

When we are working with a couple, we don't just throw in the towel if there are communication issues or ruptures in trust. We get to work in therapy and process the emotions and develop skills to work through these in between sessions. Earlier in this chapter, we learned about the concept of We-ness and communal coping. While current literature does not offer specifics on how we should approach this in couples or family counseling, there are a few recommendations provided by Rohrbaugh (2020). See Exercise 16.1 for prompts to use with couples.

These can help you work alongside the couple to help them recognize their strengths and explore potential solutions together. Each session is designed to encourage collaboration and focus on problem solving and goal setting. The therapist will be there to offer support and guidance, but it's important for the couple to take the lead in putting their ideas into action. This journey is about working together and nurturing their relationship in a meaningful way (Simran, 2023). In a manner similar to narrative therapy, the goal is to help couples draw upon their own experiences. It is important to ask them about solutions that have worked in the past and to encourage them to recall times when they successfully collaborated to overcome challenges. Clinicians will focus on addressing interpersonal difficulties that may hinder their ability to work together toward solutions. This approach may also involve individual sessions with their respective therapists.

Recommend Resources and Assistive Devices

Your clients may not be aware of assistive devices and resources that are available to them or that may be helpful. Assistive devices such as power wheelchairs, hearing aids, walkers, shower chairs, and devices for amputees are essential tools for many individuals. (And remember that you as a clinician need to be meeting the needs of your clients, so I have included a list of how you can consider those with disabilities in your own practice in Exercise 16.2.) For example, I regularly use a shower chair because it makes my life much easier. However, when I travel, I often find that many places don't have them available. A shower bench isn't quite the same, and I typically need to ask for a shower chair in advance.

Requesting help can be daunting. An individual often feels pressured to justify their needs by explaining their pain and limitations. This stress can prevent them from asking for the assistance they require. I'm guilty of this myself. There are times I push myself too hard only to end up needing help anyway.

It's crucial for everyone to understand the importance of empathy and support in these situations. While the need for assistance is clear, I find I'm less likely to ask for it if I feel the need to justify why I require help.

How I Use an Assistive Device

May 6, 2023—Let's talk about shower chairs! I first used one after my first spine surgery and I've pretty much used it almost consistently since my fusion. It's a choice and it's for comfort. I can shower without one and I do when I go away for work, but it makes things like washing my hair and shaving my legs much easier. Not having the mobility in my spine makes certain things uncomfortable in the shower, so this is something that gives me a little extra help and comfort! They are pretty inexpensive. I had my last one for several years and it was time to get rid of it and get a new one. Super easy to put together, too.

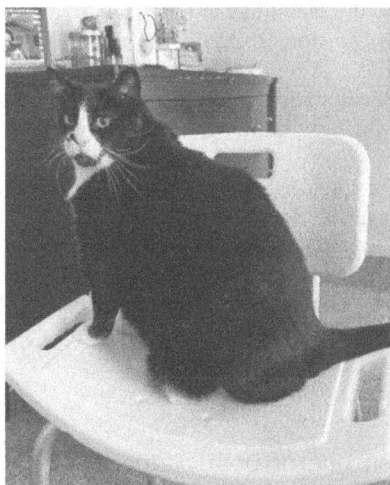

My old man and one of my emotional support cats, Rocky, loves to sit on my shower chair, every day!

Exercise 15.1: Narrative to Develop We-ness

Ask the following questions to your clients who are struggling with a chronic illness in their relationship (Rohrbaugh, 2020):

- What has been most challenging about the illness individually and as a couple?
- How are you as a couple aside from the illness?
- How did you meet?
- Do you go on dates with each other?
- How do you deal with conflict?
- What do you see as challenges for each other?
- How do you cope with these challenges?
- How do you cope as a couple?
- How does the illness interfere with or disrupt your relationship?
- Can you think of a time when you coped in communal coping, together as a couple?
- How do you feel you are doing as a team?

Exercise 15.2: Take Stock of Your Program's Level of Americans with Disabilities Act (ADA) Accessibility

This is not an exercise for you to do with a client, but this is for you as a clinician to complete about your own practice. Consider how you serve those with disabilities and how you might be able to modify your practice to better support those with visible and invisible limitations. There are standards set by the ADA, which is "a federal civil rights law that prohibits discrimination against people with disabilities in everyday activities" (U.S. Department of Justice Civil Rights Division, 2022). Ask yourself the following:

- Do you have an elevator and fully ADA-compliant bedroom and bathroom?
- If you are in an outpatient building, do you have ramps, larger chairs, and ADA facilities?
- In a treatment center setting, do you have a shower chair, toilet seat riser, and other devices available if needed?
- What can you do to improve the physical layout of your space to be accessible? (Some spaces have many ADA-compliant components but not all of them, such as wider doorways to accommodate wheelchairs.)
- What are the ADA guidelines for your facility?

Summary

In relationships, when one or both partners have a chronic illness, the illness is a third party in the relationship. Looking at it through the lens of We-ness and communal coping can lead couples to feel supported, seen, and heard. Many with chronic illnesses have suffered attachment traumas and have felt as though they have to "pay the price" for needing help from a partner. The reality is that there are some people who do not want to date someone with a chronic illness. There isn't much research on this topic, so we focused on lived experiences in this chapter, from the author as well as Agamemnon and Zephyr. This chapter offers suggestions including finding the right resources and assistive devices and solution-focused couples therapy. In our next chapter, I will examine resilience.

References

American Society for Metabolic and Bariatric Surgery. (n.d.). *Life After Bariatric Surgery*. https://asmbs.org/patients/life-after-bariatric-surgery

Attachment Project. (2023, November 15). How to heal from an attachment wound. https://www.attachmentproject.com/psychology/attachment-wound

Attachment Project. (n.d.). What is attachment trauma? www.attachmentproject.com/psychology/attachment-trauma

Davidson, E. (2024, January 10). A sick girl's guide to navigating dating with a chronic illness. CreakyJoints. https://creakyjoints.org/about-arthritis/rheumatoid-arthritis/ra-patient-perspectives/dating-chronic-illness

Gladwell, H. (2020, August 28). No, chronic illness doesn't make you a partner's burden. Healthline. www.healthline.com/health/chronic-illness/chronic-illness-does-not-make-you-a-burden#6

Rohrbaugh, M. J. (2020). Constructing We-ness: A communal coping intervention for couples facing chronic illness. *Family Process*, 60(1). https://doi.org/10.1111/famp.12595

Simran. (2023, April 1). Solution-focused couples therapy: Techniques and benefits. Mantra Care. https://mantracare.org/therapy/relationship/solution-focused-couples-therapy

U.S. Department of Justice Civil Rights Division. (2022). Introduction to the Americans with Disabilities Act. www.ada.gov/topics/intro-to-ada

Chapter 16

Resilience and Quality of Life

Resilience is a skill that can be honed and practiced and will help with eating disorder recovery, injury recovery, and life with a chronic medical condition. There are many definitions of resilience, and each person can determine what that means for them. To me, resilience is not bouncing back to some past form of myself; it is recovering to a newer version of myself. There have been and will be countless new versions of myself.

The American Psychological Association (2024) defines resilience as "the process and outcome of successfully adapting to difficult or challenging life experiences, especially through mental, emotional, and behavioral flexibility and adjustment to external and internal demands."

Many factors play a role in how well individuals cope with adversity. How we view and engage with the world around us can make a significant difference, as can the support we receive from our social networks. It's important to remember that there are various coping strategies that can help us navigate tough times. Research shows that the qualities and resources associated with resilience are not fixed; they can be cultivated and strengthened over time. With patience and practice, we can all learn to bounce back from challenges (American Psychological Association, 2024).

Relationship Between Chronic Illness and Resilience

There are many studies looking at chronic illness and resilience to understand how individuals live with and move beyond the limitations of chronic illness. For example, one systematic review looked at 12 studies involving more than 7,100 participants from diverse backgrounds, exploring important topics such as social support in diabetes management and the impact of resilience on mental health outcomes for cancer patients. The review stated: "The insights from this study align with positive psychology, emphasizing how important social resilience can be in helping individuals face the challenges that come with chronic diseases. Research in this area is still in its early stages" (Ye, 2022).

DOI: 10.4324/9781003500254-21

This review highlights an important finding: resilience plays a vital role in shaping self-care behaviors, which can influence health outcomes. It is crucial to recognize and honor the connection between resilience and the experience of living with an illness. By focusing on interventions that nurture and strengthen resilience in individuals, we can offer meaningful support that enhances their overall well-being.

The findings from this article also shed light on the challenges many face, indicating an *inverse correlation* between resilience and mental health issues such as depression, anxiety, incapacitation, and somatization. "An inverse correlation indicates a relationship between two variables where, as one variable increases, the other variable tends to decrease" (Kenton, 2019). As Cal et al. (2015) observed, "Moreover, as resilience scores increase, the progression of illness tends to decline, suggesting a hopeful path for those navigating chronic conditions. By prioritizing resilience, we can foster a more supportive environment for healing and growth."

Both/and Resiliency

In a resilient life, we are not searching for an absence of pain but instead the ability to live our lives in spite of it. With chronic illness, if we only do things when we do not feel pain or focus on our limitations, we would miss out on many life-enhancing activities. Instead, we are seeking joy and a fulfilled life in the presence of pain and illness. Both can exist.

For example, the other day, I got a text from my running friend. It was a picture of her with our running group saying that they missed me. I missed them, too, and I was a little sad that I could not run with them because I am injured. While I could not be with them, I was finding joy in other places. I did a workout to celebrate the life of an incredible woman who lost her battle with cancer. Then I got to enjoy lunch with another dear friend and then visit with yet another while sitting with the sun on my face. If that isn't happiness and joy, I don't know what is. If I had allowed myself to stay in that sadness and longing to be with my running crew, I would not have been able to experience the joy of that day where I got hugs and laughter through tears as I honored my friend with others, I enjoyed good food and the sun on my face and wind in my hair, and I got to hear the laughter of my friend's kids and enjoy a heart-to-heart catch-up.

Creating an Individual Quality of Life

Quality of life is an important factor for individuals living with chronic illness and seeking resilience. In my search for a definition of quality of life, I was not able to find one universal definition, but a common theme included "health and free from disease or illness." Obviously, for those with chronic illness, this is impossible. Individuals living with chronic illnesses need to create their own definition that acknowledges the limitations they may experience with their chronic illness while still seeking a whole life.

In my life with scoliosis, the concept of quality of life came up as I prepared for my major surgery in 2018. When Dr. Tantorski and I talked about the procedure, we discussed my quality of life. At that time, my pain was interrupting all areas of my life, and it was constant. I often canceled plans or didn't make any. My life had gotten small, and my quality of life had dwindled.

Quality of life can mean so many things to so many people. For those of us in a body that doesn't work "the way it is supposed to," we cannot afford to wait until we feel well to enjoy life. And how do we define "feeling well" anyway? We are striving toward a full life, no matter how our body feels from day to day. *The goal is to thrive and have a good quality of life, movement, self-care, and love even in the presence of pain, discomfort, and uncertainty. The focus is on the here and now.*

For me, sometimes quality of life is the joy of swinging on the rings or running outside, and other times it is snuggling with my cats while I have heat and ice on my aching parts.

Values Play a Role in our Resilience and Quality of Life

We all have different values and things that are important to us, so it is challenging to have a universal scoring system for quality of life because it is separate and distinct for all of us. One example is that for some people, having children is a strong determinant of their quality of life, while this is not a consideration for others.

My values include time with friends, supporting my community, fitness, self-care, living with purpose, authenticity, using my personal experience to help others, quality time with loved ones, animal welfare (my cats!), sobriety, independence, integrity, reliability, gratitude, advocacy, and respect for myself and others. This is not an exhaustive list; however, it is enough information for me to take a look at my life and see if I am living within my values or not. If there are areas of my life that do not align with my values, I notice them and work to improve in those areas. I can still live within these values when I am in times of health and less pain, and also when I am in times of injury, illness, or surgery recovery.

How I fit into my values will look different based on which phase of life I am in. When an individual creates their own list, they should still have these things in their life when they are in a time of more illness and limitations and anywhere on the spectrum from illness to wellness. How these values play out in their life will certainly look different based on their illness and wellness stage.

I will dig a little deeper here to fully explain. For example, when I am in a "time of illness," I am able to spend time with friends by meeting for a meal or coffee. Sometimes, instead, I might connect with them via a phone call or a text. When I am in a "time of wellness," this might look like going for a hike or going out dancing. Neither is better than the other as they are expressions of *my value of time with friends.*

Encourage individuals to create their values list, keeping in mind "times of wellness and illness". If they do not like that descriptor, they can find words that better fit their own mindset as long as they are neutral. We want to stay as neutral as possible in our words because the goal is to thrive in any stage, so we don't want to put wellness on a pedestal as the goal. The goal is quality of life, no matter where an individual is on the spectrum of health. This is different for all of us. As I see it, neutral words allow us to name the phase that we are in, such as injury, surgery recovery, or pain flare.

Another Determinant of Quality of Life Is Measured by What Brings Joy

Joy can be found in the simplest things: a favorite coffee drink, a funny meme or reel from a friend, a snuggle from a pet, and the sun on one's face. Individuals get to enjoy these things in the face of pain and limitations. When an individual is in a season where they have less pain and limitations, their joy may look different: taking a long walk, going rock climbing, seeing live music. For me and countless others, finding what brings joy is also a key.

Joy can come from the little things in life and the ability to see and notice them. When individuals are struggling with depression, anxiety, and disordered eating, this may be tough to identify. Individuals can find help from their therapist, dietitian, support group, and friends if they struggle with their mental well-being. For me, joy is waking up to a fat cat laying on my belly, grilled cheese sandwiches, seeing my friend's kids in musicals, swinging on the rings, big hugs, laughter, walking barefoot in the grass. Over time, the things that bring me joy can change, whereas my values typically stay the same.

How Can an Individual Achieve Joy in the Presence of Pain?

To experience joy, an individual needs to determine how they can achieve those things even in the presence of illness or pain. So, how does one live within their values *and* find joy, every single day, even in the midst of pain and suffering? That can mean physical or emotional or both. As I have written throughout this book, emotional pain often accompanies physical suffering. If an individual is waiting for no pain or illness to have a positive quality of life, they may be waiting forever. My intention in this book is not to make sure an individual has no discomfort or physical challenges. I wish that were the case for all of us. However, that is not the reality for many. What we can do instead is make sure we can have a happy and fulfilling life, no matter what our body is doing and feeling from day to day.

Finding a Peaceful Place

August 19, 2024—Today, I'm not defeated; I have some personal relationship challenges and I am feeling heartache. So, after time with a friend, instead of going home I drove right towards City Island; my car just went there. It was awesome to see the raging river after the crazy storms that we had.

I walked across the Walnut Street Bridge then along the waterfront to walk the Harvey Taylor Bridge. I have run and walked a lot of races there, including half marathons and the Capitol 10 Miler. I have had a lot of training runs with my running gang and they are so special to me. When I was on that bridge, I had the biggest smile on my face and even sang my music out loud to myself. It felt so good because I have so many memories of my time there. Not all of those memories are positive memories, but they are all meaningful.

The Capitol 10 Miler is the first time I had ever run 10 miles after my spine was fused. After my spine was injured by a chiropractor a few summers ago, I couldn't run but I walked in that half marathon. So, there are beautiful memories and important reminders of my resilience. There were many times when I was struggling physically and emotionally that I have gone to that bridge to walk or run with friends or on my own, and I have always felt better.

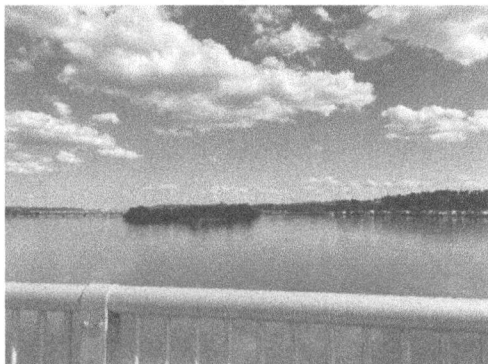

Finding a Peaceful Place

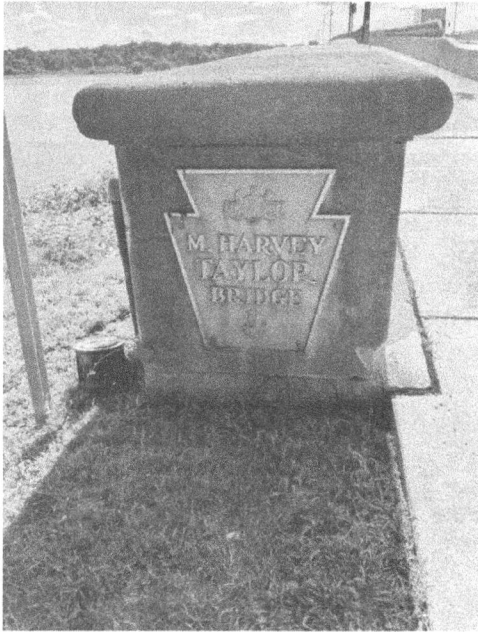

Finding a Peaceful Place

Utilizing Others to Build Resilience

A Little Help from Our Friends

When someone is in a dark time, emotionally or physically, they often need support or reminders from friends and family. An individual may not be able to ask themselves how they are going to find joy today. Instead, their people will ask and remind them. Their people can ask them how they are going to take care of themselves today, what can make them smile today, what can bring them joy today.

As a personal example, as I'm writing this, I'm having a tough day emotionally. I am feeling rejected. I reached out to friends for support. And I have decided that my joy today will come from writing, drinking coffee, seeing my friend's musical, and trying the indoor rock-climbing gym. I am still recovering from sports injuries so I may not be able to climb for long, but I will be happy to climb for ten minutes!

Who Are My People?

Some individuals may wonder, "What if I don't have 'my people'?" This can mean many things. In a chronically ill and eating-disordered life and body, their world may have gotten smaller regarding connections and finding their community. These people can be friends that an individual makes in a support group, lifelong friends, teammates, family, or chosen family.

Remind your clients to not be discouraged if they don't feel like they have their people; those people are trying to find them, too. I have met some friends through social media, work, sports, and volunteer opportunities. We can see everything as an opportunity to make a new connection. You never know who may become a close friend. Instruct an individual to take a look at all areas of their life to see where they can find friends in real life; they may already have casual connections that could turn into closer friendships. And they can also try other avenues.

Advocacy Is an Important Part of Resilience

Advocacy can mean many things to many people. It can mean advocating in the nation's capital, which I will be doing the week I write this as I advocate for important eating disorder legislation. It could mean stating one's needs to family and friends. To advocate is scary; however, it can be very empowering. An individual using their voice to ask to get their needs met is vulnerable because people can say no to what they are asking for. To take one step back, it is vulnerable for an individual to even admit that they have needs, let alone say it out loud to another person. Someone might think, "If I have needs, I might need other people. I can get hurt. I am not truly independent. I can't do it on my own."

Individuals may find reframing their thoughts and using cognitive behavioral therapy skills to be useful when they encounter thoughts like these. Go back to Chapter 13 to find some guidance.

Advocating in the Workplace

When individuals advocate for themselves in the workplace, it can often feel daunting and intimidating. When their voices aren't being heard, human resources can be a helpful resource. But keep in mind that advocating doesn't always work out despite the effort.

Personally, I experienced poor treatment from an employer due to temporary limitations after surgery. Despite working remotely for a couple of months, I performed exceptionally well in my role. My career involves travel, but with a broken wrist and clavicle, I was unable to drive or travel during that time. This situation was not well received, and it was hurtful to be treated poorly. I felt as though I was doing something wrong and that I wasn't good at my job. Given the choice, I would have preferred to be on the road all day for work rather than stuck at home, struggling to perform simple tasks like opening a bottle of water.

I reached out to friends for support and advocated for myself with my employer. Ultimately, I made the decision to leave and found a new job where I am much happier. It was difficult and painful to present my case only to have it denied. Despite many years of experience, self-advocacy continues to be a challenge for me.

Even though our needs may not always be met, an individual will likely feel empowered when they are able to ask for what they need. At times, it is still challenging to do this, and this is one of those things that a support network can help with.

When an individual is able to advocate for themselves and use their voice, it gives them more choice in their life instead of things happening "to them."

Advocating Becomes a Skill

It may never feel comfortable for an individual to advocate for themselves, but the more they ask, the more it will become a skill they can access when needed. For example, if an individual is going in for a medical appointment, advocating for themselves can look like having a list questions and not leaving until they have satisfactory answers to all of them. This is how I determined who would perform my spine surgeries. I had second (and third) opinions. My trust in my doctor increased when I sat down with my long list of questions—I had them in one of the notes on my phone—and he answered all of them. He did not rush me and responded with kindness and empathy. It is scary to trust someone, even more so when your life is literally in their hands.

Use Your Voice for Others

Another type of advocacy that has changed my life is being able to use my voice for those who are not able to use theirs. For me, that has looked like me telling my story, creating a safe space for others to tell their stories, smashing scales, advocating in my state and national capital, and becoming a part of organizations that can create change in the big picture. As I write this, I have returned home from my first professional scoliosis conference where I presented my poster on scoliosis, spine fusion, body image, and mental health. I was the only mental health provider in a space full of international medical professionals. It was important for me to be there to be a voice for so many others. I'm always happy to use my voice to help someone who cannot use their own.

Activities for Clinicians

Exercise 16.1: Reminders of Resilience

Sometimes, when an individual feels down and defeated, they need reminders of their own resilience. They need to feel when they have experienced it and felt it. This is where a clinician can help an individual identify their own personal reminders of resilience. You can ask your client the following questions:

1   Can you think of a time when you felt resilient?

   - What was the situation or event?
   - What was it about it that made you feel resilient?
   - Can you picture it in your mind?
   - Describe how it felt.

2   What is your special place where you have reminders of your resilience?

   - What happened in that place?
   - Were you alone or with someone?
   - Do you have photos for reminders?
   - Is this a place you can physically visit?
   - If not, are you able to picture it and experience it in your mind and memory?

Exercise 16.2: Examining Individual Values

The following is an activity that a clinician can use to help a client define their values. Here is a script that may be useful when working with an individual:

So the first step is to determine your values and what you define as your quality of life. You can take many online quizzes to help you choose your values. Your values may have been determined by your family, friends, community, religion, and culture. I would encourage you to stop and take this time to write them down. (Do this with your client.) Consider the following:

   - What are some non-negotiables in your life?
   - What do you need to feel joy, satisfaction, peace, and hope?

If you are stumped, you can look up long lists of values and see what resonates with you. We all have our core values: the non-negotiables, the must-haves, the things that make you "you"! If you like, you can break these down into fine minutia and distinguish values for yourself as well as your relationships, social outlets, work, financial health, religious beliefs, and so on.

Summary

Resilience is a skill that can be developed and practiced, aiding in recovery from eating disorders, rehabilitating injuries, and managing chronic medical conditions. Several factors influence how well individuals cope with adversity, including one's perspective on and engagement with the world around them as well as the support they receive from their social networks.

It's essential to remember that various coping strategies can help individuals navigate difficult times. Finding joy, living according to one's values, and engaging in advocacy are all connected to an individual's overall quality of life. It is important to identify one's values, remind oneself of one's resilience, and understand that one can lead a resilient life.

References

American Psychological Association. (2024). Resilience. www.apa.org/topics/resilience

Cal, S. F., Sá, L. R. de, Glustak, M. E., & Santiago, M. B. (2015). Resilience in chronic diseases: A systematic review. *Cogent Psychology*, *2*(1). https://doi.org/10.1080/23311908.2015.1024928

Kenton, W. (2019). What inverse correlation tells us. Investopedia. www.investopedia.com/terms/i/inverse-correlation.asp

Ye, Z. J. (2022). Editorial: Resilience in chronic disease. *Frontiers in Psychiatry, 13*. https://doi.org/10.3389/fpsyt.2022.846370

Final Thoughts

Finding Peace

In the final chapter, I mentioned walking at City Island, my reminder of resilience. I also mentioned a friend and how she reached out to me. This morning, I met her at City Island for a chilly walk with friends followed by brunch. I knew that I would no longer be running there.

The most recent recommendation from my doctor is to no longer run based on my new spine images. A couple of weeks ago, I went through all of the stages of grief after getting this news. I was sad. *Why did I have to lose one more thing?* I did not want to talk to anyone about it because I didn't think they would understand. I felt fear of the future. I felt angry. I couldn't say the words out loud without crying. My grief was not about the sport so much as the fear of the loss of community. The last time I ran there, I ran a race with my friend by my side, walking, jogging, and laughing. At that time, I didn't know that it would be my last run. Now I'm happy that it was because I have amazing memories of that day.

As we walked City Island this morning, I felt at peace.

Our Journey Together

This book took you on a journey through my story and the unique lived experiences of several others. My intention and hope is that you were able to learn through the stories in addition to the research and practical applications. If you are a client, I hope you felt seen and heard and not alone. I hope you were able to connect to these lived experiences. May they bring you strength in your struggle and may you know that you are never alone. You can live a life with joy and resilience in the presence of pain.

Summary

Chronic Illness and Chronic Pain

A chronic illness can be either congenital or acquired later in life and is classified as chronic if it lasts more than one year. There is a known link

DOI: 10.4324/9781003500254-22

between chronic illnesses and eating disorders, but research in this area is limited. Diet-related chronic conditions may have a higher occurrence of disordered eating. The emotional impact of chronic illness can disrupt a person's sense of self, potentially leading to mental health issues, including eating disorders. We can help clients redefine their illness, allowing it to become part of their identity rather than defining it.

Chronic pain lasts three months or longer and is the primary reason people seek medical care. Since pain is subjective, individual experiences vary, and it's important to ask questions to gauge this. Chronic pain can lead to stress and is a risk factor for suicidal thoughts. As part of routine assessments, clinicians and other health providers should evaluate clients for eating disorder symptoms, pain levels, and suicidal ideation. Clients with a high pain threshold may ignore critical danger signals. Collaborate with clients to establish a management plan for pain flare-ups that includes both physical and emotional support.

Inner Critic Development

The words we hear about ourselves in childhood shape our inner critic. A diagnosis of illness at a young age can lead to a loss of self-identity. Support and discussion around body image are crucial upon receiving a medical diagnosis and as the illness progresses.

Self-objectification and social comparison are common but can trigger eating disorders, especially in those whose bodies are affected by illness or disability. It's important to differentiate between body image disturbance related to illness and distortion associated with eating disorders, and to assess both together.

Using neutral language can help address these challenges, and various questionnaires can effectively measure changes in body image and quality of life concerning illness.

Invisible Disability

Invisible disabilities lack obvious signs of illness. Static disabilities remain unchanged, while dynamic disabilities fluctuate in abilities and pain levels. People with chronic illnesses may exhibit hyper-independence, making it hard to seek help. Encouraging interdependence can enhance independence by fostering mutual support in relationships. Individuals can cultivate interdependence through individual and group therapy.

Grief

Grief is complicated, particularly for those with lifelong illnesses. It encompasses various aspects such as career, future, abilities, and relationships.

Support is essential during this process, as denial can hinder seeking medical attention. Individuals may need help from therapists and loved ones to navigate their changing roles and identities. JK's experience highlights the importance of recognizing grief and utilizing support systems to manage daily life. Staying present can help mitigate fears about the future.

Presurgical Mental Health

Presurgical psychological testing can identify potential mental health issues after surgery, allowing for better preparation. Pre-existing depression and anxiety can lead to complications and increased pain. Medical providers should screen for these conditions and work with the patient's therapist. Clinicians can help clients prepare using SMART goals, cognitive behavioral therapy (CBT), mindfulness techniques, and assessing mitigating factors.

Medical Trauma and Weight Stigma

The psychosocial stages of development highlight how chronic illnesses diagnosed in childhood affects individuals throughout their lives. Medical trauma can arise in healthcare settings, potentially leading to medical traumatic stress or PTSD. Clinicians can use various screening tools to assess and plan treatment for those impacted.

Weight stigma in the medical system often results in patients not following medical advice, avoiding appointments, or neglecting essential care. This bias can lead to disordered eating or relapse in those with a history of eating disorders. Recent studies show that presurgical weight loss may be harmful. While more research on weight management in chronic illness is necessary, patients frequently face weight assessments at appointments, so it's crucial to prepare them.

For healing, bodies need both energy and rest. Dietitians play a key role in helping clients develop meal plans that accommodate periods of illness, wellness, and surgery.

Treatment Modalities

As clinicians, we use various treatment modalities to address trauma and eating disorders. Establishing safety and containment with clients is crucial before starting trauma work. Effective methods include narrative therapy, play therapy, EMDR, acceptance and commitment therapy, and progressive desensitization, which can help with body image issues from illness, injury, or surgery. Play therapy is particularly effective for children with medical trauma or PTSD.

Therapeutic Alliance

A strong therapeutic alliance and relationship-focused care lead to better outcomes. I compared the relationship in physical therapy to dating to emphasize its importance. As clinicians, we advocate for our clients and collaborate with their medical teams, bridging the educational gap by informing providers about eating disorders. We also prepare clients to find suitable medical providers and guide them throughout their journey.

Sports Injury Psychology

Sports injury psychology provides valuable insights for working with clients who have eating disorders and chronic illnesses. Community and social support are crucial for these groups. Clients often fear returning to work, school, or sports after setbacks. Recovery from an injury, eating disorder, or surgery can lead to positive life changes beyond the immediate recovery. As clinicians, we can assist clients by helping them change their narratives and set realistic SMART goals.

Those with chronic illnesses often relate to the spoon theory, a helpful framework for discussing pain and energy reserves. Understanding this can aid clinicians in conversations about these experiences. The DSM-5 recognizes Illness Related Anxiety, or Health Anxiety, and CBT is particularly effective for managing anxiety related to health changes or increased pain. Finding neutral thoughts can also help process feelings about ongoing health shifts and future fears.

Movement Is Medicine

Movement has physical and emotional benefits, but it requires caution and intention for those with chronic illnesses and eating disorders. While movement can sometimes be joyful, it is also essential for rehabilitation after an injury. For individuals recovering from eating disorders, returning to sports is possible with proper planning, support, and engaged, embodied movement.

Fear of movement can hinder recovery, but it can be overcome. Clinicians should avoid demonizing exercise or creating fear around movement. It's crucial to meet clients where they are and facilitate healthy, body-grounded movement.

Relationships and Resilience

In relationships affected by chronic illness, the illness often becomes a third party. Emphasizing "We-ness" and communal coping helps couples feel supported and understood. Many individuals with chronic illnesses face attachment traumas and may feel guilty for needing support.

Resilience is a skill that can be developed, helping with recovery from eating disorders, injuries, and chronic medical conditions. How well we cope with adversity depends on our mindset and the support from our social networks.

Various coping strategies can help us through tough times. Focusing on joy, living by our values, and advocating for causes we care about can improve our quality of life.

How Can Clinicians Better Serve This Population

It's crucial to understand that you don't have to have experienced the same challenges as your client to provide meaningful support. While many clinicians specializing in eating disorders have their own recovery stories, it's not a requirement to effectively help others in need. The same goes for those dealing with chronic illnesses.

Chronic illnesses can be part of the perfect storm that creates an eating disorder, so we need to be sure to include this in our history taking. A chronic illness can make an eating disorder exponentially more challenging to treat due to medical complications, body image disturbance, and lack of understanding. Our clients with eating disorders are intuitive and resilient and, with your help and understanding, can live with a chronic illness and achieve full recovery from their eating disorder.

Take the time to connect with your clients on a deeper level—listen to their stories, learn from their experiences, and do your own research to better understand their condition. Creating a safe and welcoming space, where they feel valued and heard, is vital. Approach this work with curiosity and openness, and don't hesitate to share what you've learned along the way. Above all, strive to make your environments accessible to everyone, ensuring that all feel supported and included.

Connect with Me

If this book has made a positive impact on you, I would genuinely love to hear your thoughts. If you find yourself needing more support, please don't hesitate to reach out.

Instagram: @authortamiegangloff
Facebook: Author Tamie Gangloff
Website: www.tamiegangloff.com

Index

For Product Safety Concerns and Information please contact our EU
representative GPSR@taylorandfrancis.com
Taylor & Francis Verlag GmbH, Kaufingerstraße 24, 80331 München, Germany